the Black death
the Impact of the
fourteenth-Century plague

medieval & renaissance texts & studies

VOLUME 13

the Black Death
the Impact of the
fourteenth-Century plague

Papers of the Eleventh Annual Conference
of the Center for Medieval & Early Renaissance Studies

EDITED BY

Daniel Williman

INTRODUCTION BY

Nancy Siraisi

medieval & Renaissance texts & studies
Center for Medieval & Early Renaissance Studies
Binghamton, New York
1982

Library of Congress Cataloging in Publication

State University of New York at Binghamton. Center for
Medieval and Early Renaissance Studies. Conference (11th :
1977)
    The black death: the impact of the fourteenth-century
plague.

    (Medieval & Renaissance texts & studies; 13)
    Contents: The black death: the crisis and its social and
economic consequences / by J. M. W. Bean — The plague
as key to meaning in Boccaccio's Decameron / by Aldo S.
Bernardo — Al-Manbiji's Report of the plague: a treatise on
the plague of 764-65/1362-64 / by Michael Dols — [etc.]
    1. Black death—Congresses. 2. Civilization, Medieval—
Congresses. I. Williman, Daniel. II. Title. III. Series:
Medieval & Renaissance texts & studies; 13.
RC171.S8   1977   940.1'92   82-12435
ISBN 0-86698-050-4

Printed in the United States of America

Contents

pReface

The Center for Medieval and Early Renaissance Studies has traditionally chosen the topics of its annual conferences from among the literally crucial questions raised by the events of these epochs, questions that can serve as crossroads for the largest number and greatest variety of scholars. The Black Death, the surprising visitation of plague in 1348, followed by successive epidemic waves until the seventeenth century, was thus a natural choice for the Eleventh Conference, which took place on October 21–23, 1977.

The scholars who came to show their findings and ask their questions, from their studies of medicine, society, literature and art, made the meeting a vigorous and profitable exchange. This volume contains articles by six conferees, rewritten for print and in part revised in the light of insights derived from that weekend, together with an Introduction derived from the state-of-the-question report that Professor Nancy Siraisi offered on the last morning of the meeting.

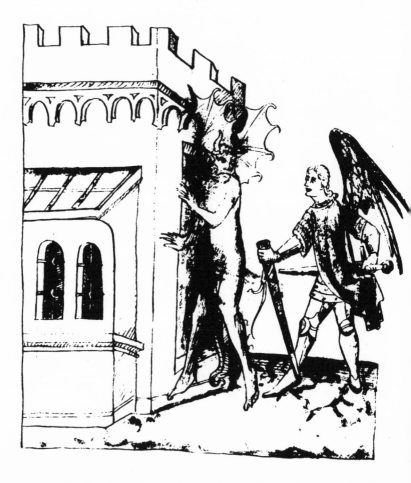

An angel binding Satan for one thousand years, from Telesphorus, *Libellus de causis, statu, cognitione ac fine scismatis et tribulationum futurarum,* written toward the end of the fourteenth century. The illumination is reproduced from Munich, Bayerische Staatsbibliothek, MS Clm 313, f. 28v, executed shortly after 1431 in or around Salzburg.

Introduction[1]

Nancy Siraisi

For contemporary chroniclers, the plague pandemic of 1347–1350 was one of the worst disasters ever to afflict the human race — an estimate that has, as Robert Lerner reminds us in one of the essays collected in the present volume, been echoed in more recent times.[2] Furthermore, the tragic events of those years marked the opening of a period of almost four centuries in which Europe and the Middle East were to be struck by repeated outbreaks of the same disease. If by the seventeenth and eighteenth centuries plague epidemics no longer swept across Europe, they could nonetheless still have a catastrophic, if temporary, effect on the life of major cities: London in 1665, Marseilles in 1720. Unavoidably, any general analysis of the culture and society of the Later Middle Ages must take account of the first impact of this, as it then appeared, new and uncontrollable force in human affairs.

The subject of plague in Europe in the late Middle Ages has certainly not been neglected either by writers contemporary with the first great outbreaks or by their successors in the nineteenth and twentieth centuries. In particular, the great epidemic of the mid-fourteenth century has long been recognized not only as a human calamity with few parallels in recorded history, but also as a factor in the subsequent social, economic, religious, and cultural development of medieval Europe. Despite the copiousness of the historical literature on the Black Death, as the first fourteenth-century epidemic came later to be called, the overall impact on society of that dreadful visitation remains curiously ill-defined. Even such basic questions as the extent and distribution of plague mortality are still vigorously debated, so that it is hardly surprising that no satisfactory consensus has been reached on such complex issues as the specific effects of plague on the economy or on that amorphous entity, the consciousness of the age. One can readily appreciate the decision of the author of a recent survey of fourteenth-century history who tells us that she initially set out to identify the effects of plague on society but, since "the question . . . escaped an answer," turned to a different approach.[3]

Yet one must admit to a certain puzzlement at this situation. How can the effects of so dire a calamity be so hard to synthesize satisfactorily? Numerous sources are available and many of them have been carefully examined. The dramatic interest of what B. G. Babington, who was stimulated by the cholera outbreaks of his own day to produce an English translation (1844) of Hecker's pioneer work on medieval epidemics, termed "a convulsion of the human race, unequalled in violence and extent,"[4] ensured the early identification and, where necessary, the printing of almost all the major contemporary narrative, literary, and medical descriptions of the plague of 1347–50 as it appeared in western Europe. Moreover, since the latter part of the nineteenth century local archival records of various kinds have been combed to provide the basis for numerous detailed studies of the impact of plague on particular western European cities, regions, and countries, as well as institutions and professions.[5] While, as will become apparent from what follows, much basic research remains to be done, much has already been accomplished.

The obstacles that have, nonetheless, hitherto hindered the construction of any satisfactory general analysis on the basis of these sources and studies have been, I believe, of four principal kinds. The first of these has to do with the state of medical and biological knowledge of the disease itself. Modern historical understanding of the plague in Europe is to a significant extent the child of the scientific understanding of the disease achieved since the identification of the plague bacillus in 1894 and the treatment of late nineteenth- and early twentieth-century outbreaks of plague in India and elsewhere. Yet the integration of developments in scientific knowledge of plague with the historical picture is neither a simple task nor one that can be regarded as capable of being accomplished once and for all. On the contrary, the task of making historical sense by simultaneously taking into consideration both the records of the past and the current achievements of rapidly evolving disciplines — in this instance biology and medicine — is, and is likely to remain, a complex and challenging one. As R. S. Roberts has pointed out,[6] the historian must be aware of the scientific short-comings not only of his primary but also of many of his secondary sources. Thus Creighton, the author of a still esteemed *History of Epidemics* first published in the 1890s,[7] never accepted the idea of bacterial causation and transmission of disease; his beliefs in this regard affected his selection and understanding of the data provided by early chronicles and records. At the same time, excessive reliance upon medical and demographic accounts of fairly recent outbreaks of plague in, say, India, is also hazardous, since over a period of time the behavior and virulence of disease bacteria may also change without any deliberate human intervention.

Secondly, our knowledge of medieval demography remains very inadequate, and understanding of any or all aspects of the role of plague in medieval society must rest at bottom upon an evaluation of the demographic significance of the disease. This is obviously true of hypotheses about the social and economic effects of plague, which depend directly on arguments about the death rate, case mortality, and distribution of mortality by age, sex, and class, and the rate of replacement of the population. The cultural impact of plague is less directly linked to demography since, presumably, events may produce an emotional response either disproportionately greater or disproportionately lesser than their actual effects, measured in statistical terms, appear to warrant. Nonetheless, one cannot suppose that the cultural reaction, or lack of reaction, to plague was totally unrelated to plague mortality. But the data concerning population trends which are found in or can be derived from fourteenth-century records are, for the most part, too few, too scattered, and too random both in their original formulation and their survival, to allow any satisfactory large-scale synthesis, although, as was already noted, highly useful small-scale studies of particular towns, religious communities, professions, and so on, continue to accumulate. For the larger picture, however, the historian is frequently thrown back on plague as a biological phenomenon, a situation which, as we have just seen, presents its own problems.

The third reason why it has proved so hard to reach any consensus on the historical impact of the so-called Black Death has to do with our interpretation of the economic history of the fourteenth century. For a generation now, many historians have held that the fourteenth century was, on the whole, a period of grave economic crisis for much of Europe.[8] Numerous detailed studies have examined particular economic aspects of the century; however, the broad questions of the effect of economic trends upon institutions such as the manor and serfdom in northern Europe, as well as upon such sociological phenomena as social unrest, the growth of early Renaissance culture in Italy, and the crisis of the Church have not yet received wholly definite answers. Obviously, plague played a part in the general picture of falling population, falling productivity, and social upheaval. Identifying that part, and distinguishing the effects of plague from those of war, failures of the food supply, monetary manipulations, and class hostility, prove to be tasks of great complexity.

And fourthly, and perhaps most importantly, we are faced with the need for a new, more nuanced interpretation of the cultural effects of the Black Death in the light of current work on the intellectual and spiritual life of the later Middle Ages. In 1978, a leading specialist in the field found it appropriate to entitle an essay "Fourteenth-Century Religious Thought: A Premature Profile."[9] Nonetheless, it does not seem "premature" to say that over the last generation or so the work of historians of philosophy, theology, and science has produced a greatly improved understanding and a much more positive evaluation of aspects of late medieval culture that were formerly neglected, misunderstood, and sometimes even scorned. This re-evaluation frequently stresses both links with the past (such as the roots of late medieval mysticism in the twelfth century and, for that matter, in the patristic age) and the connections among movements formerly conceived of as more or less disparate (such as nominalism, humanism, and demands for religious reform).[10] This re-evaluation of the high culture of the age means that truisms about the impact of the Black Death upon intellectual and spiritual life also must be re-examined. So long as the thought of the late Middle Ages could be dismissed as, at best, a falling off from the achievements of the thirteenth century, or, at worst, an arid waste of decadent scholasticism, and so long as its religiosity could be characterized as notable chiefly for a morbid obsession with physical decay, then the Black Death could reasonably be called upon to account for a lasting decline in academic life, and for the emergence of a profoundly pessimistic climate of religious opinion.[11] Recent work suggests, however, that although the plague killed some scholars and professional men, its direct impact upon institutions of higher learning has been exaggerated considerably.[12] Similarly, if the religiosity of the later Middle

Ages is perceived as both linked to the traditions of the twelfth and thirteenth centuries and as, for the most part, relatively creative and optimistic, then it is less easy to see it as a long-term response to disaster. Once again, it is self-evident that the plague must have had an impact; but it requires careful work to delimit that impact and determine what form it took.

Despite these problems, the last thirty or forty years have seen great advances in the understanding of the role of plague in European history. One may note, for example, the publication in 1954 of Pollitzer's standard work summing up current knowledge of the disease itself and of its historical occurrences.[13] In the 1940s and 1950s the controversy about the economic effects of plague on later medieval society, especially in England, began with the work of Postan and Saltmarsh.[14] Millard Meiss's seminal study of the impact of the plague upon Italian religious and artistic sensibility appeared in 1951.[15] The work done in the 1940s and 1950s rapidly came to constitute a new orthodoxy, but an orthodoxy that has been subject to continual further exploration, challenge, and revision, especially in the last decade or so.

Recent studies have dealt with the epidemiology of plague and the changing patterns of the disease itself. Shrewsbury's volume on plague in the British Isles — the work of a bacteriologist, not a historian — is likely to remain standard for some time, despite the highly controversial nature of some of its conclusions.[16] Since Shrewsbury believes that medieval and early modern outbreaks of plague in Europe seldom involved the usually fatal pneumonic form of the disease, he postulates a death rate for the Black Death and for subsequent major outbreaks dramatically lower than that usually accepted by historians. Plague also receives a good deal of attention in McNeill's attempt to chart the relationship between the ravages of epidemic disease in hitherto unexposed populations and major historical events and trends.[17] In McNeill's presentation, human activities such as wars and colonization combined with the evolution, multiplication, and spread of disease organisms to form an ecology for man which was, until the mid-nineteenth century, almost completely unaffected by any deliberate human intervention in the shape of effective medical treatment and sanitary regulations.

Thus, the problems of the causes triggering the appearance, spread, and disappearance of epidemic plague in medieval and early modern Europe continue to hold attention. Jean-Noël Biraben, in a recent synthesis of the history of plague in Europe, the most comprehensive yet available, lists explanations for outbreaks of plague advanced at various times; these range from the theory of the influence of planetary conjunctions, maintained by learned men in the fourteenth century, to twentieth-century attempts to chart a relationship between sunspots and the life cycles of the colonies of wild rodents which constitute the permanent reservoirs of plague.[18] Today, about all that can be asserted with any confidence is that this disease, always present among certain rodents and carried by their parasites, has from time to time massively affected human populations, and that its transmission through those populations has been modified by climatic factors, as well as by such human activities as migration, war, and commerce. Some writers have also been inclined to hypothesize a role for human fleas and lice, as well as rat fleas, in the spread of plague epidemics in man.[19]

The reasons for the disappearance of plague from Europe in early modern times remain as much debated as those for its appearance there in the sixth century (the so-called Plague of Justinian) and again in the fourteenth. No longer is the replacement of the black rat by the brown regarded as of much significance. Instead, some modern research has indicated the possibility that immunity to plague may develop among human populations, either through exposure to related bacteria or among particular blood groups; rats too, have been observed to have developed immunity to plague in certain twentieth-century Indian outbreaks. Similar factors may have affected the historical course of the disease.[20] Nor is there agreement even as regards the role of deliberate or inadvertent human intervention in ending the series of European and Middle Eastern epidemics of which the Black Death was the first. McNeill, as already noted, wholly discounts the importance of deliberate intervention. A wealth of supporting evidence (derived, however, from a study of the patterns of other diseases at a later date) is provided for this view by the work of the medical historian and demographer Thomas McKeown who denies both that any medical or sanitary measures had any discernible effect on disease patterns before about 1870, and that any single disease could in and of itself have had a major and *long term* impact on population trends.[21] Yet Biraben suggests that the development of quarantine regulations played a significant part in ending epidemic plague both in Europe in the late seventeenth and early eighteenth centuries and at a later date in North Africa. Carlo Cipolla, who has made a careful study of such regulations in Tuscany in the sixteenth and seventeenth centuries, apparently believes that they may have had some beneficial effect, although his endorsement is framed in extremely cautious and hesitant terms.[22]

Medievalists have begun to explore hitherto untapped local records for demographic and social information. In particular, William Bowsky, Elisabeth Carpentier, and David Herlihy have been pioneers in the exploration of the rich archival resources of the Italian cities in this regard.[23] Highly significant is the beginning of investigation of the history of plague in hitherto neglected geographical areas: for example, the work of Michael Dols on the Middle East[24] and of Lawrence Langer on Russia.[25] Moreover, a start has been made in the use of twentieth-century technology for demographic studies; thus, computerization made feasible Robert S. Gottfried's study of the mortality patterns revealed in 20,000 fifteenth-century East Anglian wills.[26] (Theoretically, of course, this kind of analysis could be applied to all surviving testamentary — or other relevant — documents of the later Middle Ages. In reality, however, it must be admitted that the enormous patience demanded by such research, even when undertaken with the aid of several collaborators as well as of the computer, probably means that studies of this kind will always be limited in number and that their scope, even if larger than that of most earlier quantitative analyses in this area, will always be relatively restricted. Besides, no technological advances can solve the problem of scatter and randomness in the original records or rationalize the accidents of their survival.)

The task of evaluating, and where necessary re-evaluating, the cultural and psychological effects of plague is also being tackled by medievalists, although work embodying the newer approaches to this problem is only now beginning to appear in print. One of the most striking features of the Conference on the Black Death sponsored by the Center for Medieval and Early Renaissance Studies of the State University of New York at Binghamton in October, 1977, was the extent of the interest evinced in this aspect of the subject. Fifteen of thirty papers offered at that conference dealt with responses to the plague in art and literature; three concerned the treatment of plague by preachers or devotional authors (Christian and Muslim); seven treated of general social or sociocultural responses (the persecution of the Jews, the possible development of peasant solidarity, the growth of burial fraternities, and the appearance of quarantine regulations being some examples). By way of contrast, only four papers dealt primarily and in any detail with the distribution of mortality by region, age, sex, and class; only one with direct economic impact (upon prices); and only one with the medical understanding of plague by fourteenth-century physicians.

The papers in this volume offer the reader a representative selection of current approaches to the economic, social, and cultural consequences of the Black Death for the late medieval world. In some respects, the six essays collected here vary widely. Sources range from an unpublished Arabic plague treatise to the *Decameron*; approaches from the economic to the psycho-historical; regional focus from England to the Middle East. Yet significant common themes emerge; indeed, the very disparity of the material on which the authors draw serves to make their conclusions mutually reinforcing.

Thus, in different ways, the essays by Malcolm Bean and Michael Dols both remind us of the need for careful study of regional variations in the impact of plague. The former notes that both contemporary chronicles and modern studies of the demographic and economic consequences of plague in different localities reveal that its attack was very uneven. While further detailed regional and comparative studies are necessary, much of the range can be accounted for, as Bean shows, by drawing upon modern medical knowledge of seasonal variations in the prevalence of different types of plague, with their differing mortality rates. Thus, the author stresses that the much-discussed English evidence is by no means necessarily typical of Europe as a whole. As far as England is concerned, however, he views with some skepticism attempts to revise downward the traditionally accepted mortality rate of about 30 per cent in the first great epidemic and to minimize its economic impact.

Michael Dols has been a pioneer in investigating the history of plague in the Middle East, and he here turns to an analysis of one of the few surviving fourteenth-century Arabic plague treatises. Dols' work breaks away from the traditional western European emphasis of most studies of plague in the Middle Ages, and serves to call our attention in this context to the interaction between, and common experiences of, medieval Muslim and Christian cultures, and to the essential unity of the Mediterranean world in the period.

The remaining essays in the volume all relate to the cultural impact of the plague, and all of them imply that this impact was neither as far-reaching nor as dramatic as is often presumed to have been the case. Siegfried Wenzel examines verses on death found in sermon collections and notes little distinction in imagery or in intensity of feeling between those produced before and those written after the great epidemic. Robert Lerner investigates a number of scattered manuscript prophecies which point to an essentially similar conclusion: mid-fourteenth-century prophecies belonged to an already well established prophetic tradition; they were intended not to inspire the final collapse (or overthrow) of the existing social order, but to reassure their readers that even the chaos brought by plague was but one feature of the plan of Divine Providence, which continued to rule all things for their ultimate good. Joseph Polzer presents the case for redating the dramatic presentations of physical decay in the frescoes of the Campo Santo at Pisa before the Black Death and reminds us that the fully evolved Dance of Death long postdates it.

Perhaps the truth of the matter is that both the harsher realities of medieval life, even in such relatively good times as the twelfth and thirteenth centuries — high infant mortality, extensive malnutrition among the poor, ineffective therapeutics — and the teachings of Christian tradition on the transitoriness of human life had combined long before 1347 to provide people with very adequate psychological and cultural mechanisms for dealing with the shock and horror produced by sudden death from foul and unexplainable disease. The magnitude of the disaster of 1347–1350 surely brought these mechanisms into vigorous play; but they did not have to be newly created because they already existed. How well they functioned under stress is indicated by studies showing that particular communities recovered rapidly from the social and administrative dislocation produced by the shock of the first great plague outbreak, and that fourteenth-century public officials responded with faith, not only in religious remedies, but also in their own powers to chart humanly protective policies. This is apparently true even of the Florentines, whose response Boccaccio portrayed in very different terms.[27]

None of the foregoing should be taken to imply that the men and women of the fourteenth century were indifferent to calamity, although, as Robert Lerner has suggested (at the CEMERS panel discussion), it would be worth investigating whether or not the Black Death was generally regarded as a worse disaster than such setbacks for Christendom as the loss of the Holy Land or the outbreak of the Great Schism. The accounts of the chroniclers are, nonetheless, abundant evidence of contemporary anguish over the Black Death; yet existing modes of thought and expression provided ways of venting and coping with that anguish. That this process could, however, be a highly creative and innovative one in the hands of gifted artists is well illustrated by Aldo Bernardo's essay on Boccaccio's use of the Black Death in the *Decameron*, where, in Bernardo's view, the plague served as a constant reminder in the background of the precariousness of human life and the all-pervasive presence of evil in the world and in ourselves. The somewhat uninspired truisms of the sermon verses are in the *Decameron* transmuted into the subtler and more profound truths of a major literary work, but Boccaccio is part of the same moral universe as Friar John Grimestone and the other preachers discussed in Wenzel's essay.

It is to be hoped that the reader of this volume will come away with the conviction that the last word on plague in the Middle Ages has not yet been said. Even as regards Europe itself, the geographic focus of historical study has so far been mainly confined to the British Isles, France, Italy, and parts of Germany. Only now are a few pioneers beginning to work with Scandinavian, Iberian, or eastern European or Middle Eastern materials. But the lacunae are not solely geographic. Some particular directions for further research were pointed out by the authors of the essays presented here at a panel discussion held on the last day of the CEMERS Conference on the Black Death, and they were unanimous in the view that much work is needed in almost every area. Thus, Malcolm Bean noted that, with reference to the plague as a factor in economic history, more is known for England than for most parts of the Continent, more for France than for Germany, and more for Germany than for any area of eastern Europe. Yet even in England further investigations of manorial accounts are needed for a fuller understanding of the relation of plague outbreaks to fluctuations in agrarian revenues and agricultural prices and wages. Similarly, English wills (which do not survive in any quantity from before about 1375) and Continental notarial records may be expected to yield information about the effects of the Black Death and later plague outbreaks on personal wealth, but remain largely unexamined in this connection. Michael Dols remarked on the very great need for studies of plague in the Byzantine Empire and, especially, in medieval and early modern India and China. As far as the Muslim world is concerned, some work is being done on plague from the seventeenth to the nineteenth centuries,[28] but the earlier period has attracted little attention, while such a basic need as the cataloguing of medieval Islamic medical manuscripts has only recently been fulfilled.[29] Robert Lerner and Siegfried Wenzel both called attention to the magnitude of the mass of unpublished and unexamined prophetic and sermonic literature, respectively, analysis of which might be expected to add to our knowledge of cultural responses to the plague experience. In his turn, Aldo Bernardo observed that little is known of the reaction of humanists other than Petrarch and Boccaccio to the plague, and pointed out that it is only very recently that literary historians have begun to take seriously the moral implications of the presence of plague in the works of those two authors themselves.

This volume, then, should be read as an interim report on the state of Black Death studies. The current consensus seems to be that the massive plague outbreaks of the fourteenth century no doubt accelerated existing social, economic, and cultural trends, but neither created nor radically changed them; and that the apparent ability of late medieval society to adapt to and absorb such a major catastrophe without collapse is a remarkable tribute to the resilience of the culture. We have just seen that much work in which this thesis can be tested is waiting to be done. The present collection will have served a good purpose if it stimulates some of the further studies that are needed before we can fully evaluate the historical consequences of the Black Death.

NANCY G. SIRAISI

Hunter College of
the City University of New York

notes

1. An earlier version of this essay was developed in light of numerous discussions with Professor Bert Hansen, now of the University of Toronto, whose assistance I wish most gratefully to acknowledge.
2. See p. 77 below.
3. Barbara W. Tuchman, *A Distant Mirror: The Calamitous 14th Century* (New York, 1978), p. xiii.
4. Translator's preface to Justus F. C. Hecker, *The Black Death, Epidemics of the Middle Ages,* 1 (1859; reprint ed., Lawrence, Kansas, 1972).
5. A very extensive bibliography is contained in Jean-Noël Biraben, *Les hommes et la peste en France et dans les pays européens et méditerranéens,* 2 vols., Civilisations et Sociétés, vols. 35, 36 (1975-76), 2, pp. 186-413.
6. R. S. Roberts, "The Use of Literary and Documentary Evidence in the History of Medicine," Edwin Clarke, ed., *Modern Methods in the History of Medicine* (London, 1971), pp. 38-43.
7. Charles Creighton, *A History of Epidemics from A.D. 664 to the Extinction of the Plague,* 2 vols. (Cambridge, 1891-1894; new edition, London, 1965).
8. The bibliography on this topic is very large. A concise summary of the thesis, and bibliography, is provided in Harry A. Miskimin, *The Economy of Early Renaissance Europe, 1300-1460* (Englewood Cliffs, N.J., 1969).
9. Heiko A. Oberman, "Fourteenth-Century Religious Thought: A Premature Profile," *Speculum* 53 (1978):80-93.
10. See, for example, William J. Courtenay, "Nominalism and Late Medieval Religion," Charles Trinkaus and Heiko A. Oberman, eds., *The Pursuit of Holiness in Late Medieval and Renaissance Religion* (Leiden, 1974), pp. 26-59, and F. Edward Cranz, "Cusanus, Luther, and the Mystical Tradition," in the same volume, pp. 93-102. A notion of the current recognition of the contributions of later fourteenth- and fifteenth-century scientific writers may be gained from a survey of the excerpts from authors of that period included in Edward Grant, ed., *A Source Book in Medieval Science* (Cambridge, Mass., 1974).
11. While such interpretations are no longer often found in recent specialized works on later medieval thought, they are still, it seems, quite frequently assumed as part of the background in more general works or works on other aspects of the period. See, for example, Chap. 17, "The Effects on the Church and Man's Mind," in one of the best available summary accounts of plague in the fourteenth century, Philip Ziegler, *The Black Death* (New York, 1969).
12. See William J. Courtenay, "The Effect of the Black Death on English Higher Education," *Speculum* 55 (1980):696-714.
13. R. Pollitzer, *Plague,* World Health Organization, Monograph Series, no. 22 (Geneva, 1954).

14. John Saltmarsh, "Plague and Economic Decline in England in the Later Middle Ages," *The Cambridge Historical Journal* 7 (1941–43): 23–41, and bibliography there cited. See also J. M. W. Bean, "Plague, Population and Economic Decline in England in the Later Middle Ages," *Economic History Review*, 2d ser., 15 (1962–3), pp. 423–37, and A. S. Bridbury, "The Black Death," ibid., 26 (1973), pp. 577–92.

15. Millard Meiss, *Painting in Florence and Siena After the Black Death* (Princeton, N.J., 1951).

16. J. F. D. Shrewsbury, *A History of Bubonic Plague in the British Isles* (Cambridge, 1970). Shrewsbury's views are contested in Christopher Morris, "The Plague in Britain," *The Historical Journal* 14 (1971):205–15.

17. William H. McNeill, *Plagues and Peoples* (New York, 1976).

18. Biraben, *Les hommes et la peste*, 1, pp. 133–34, 154; 2, pp. 9–11.

19. Concerning the location of the rodent plague foci from which the Black Death originated, see also John Norris, "East or West? The Geographic Origin of the Black Death," *Bulletin of the History of Medicine* 51 (1977):1–24, and the comment by Michael Dols, ibid., 52 (1978):112–13 and response by Norris, ibid.:114–20. Norris stresses the inadequacy of the hypothesis concerning human parasites as an explanation for the great historical epidemics.

20. Biraben, *Les hommes et la peste*, 1, pp. 17–20; and, on immunity among rats, Christopher Morris, "The Plague in Britain," *The Historical Journal* 14 (1971):209. (I am grateful to Professor Dols for calling my attention to this point.)

21. McKeown's views are summarized in his article, "Medical Issues in Historical Demography," in Edwin Clarke, *Modern Methods in the History of Medicine* (London, 1971), pp. 57–74.

22. Biraben, *Les hommes et la peste*, 2, pp. 174–5; Carlo M. Cipolla, *Public Health and the Medical Profession in the Renaissance* (Cambridge, 1976), pp. 60–65.

23. William B. Bowsky, "The Impact of the Black Death upon Sienese Government and Society," *Speculum* 39 (1964):1–34; Elisabeth Carpentier, *Une ville devant la peste: Orvieto et la Peste Noire de 1348* (Paris, 1962); David Herlihy, "Population, Plague and Social Change in Rural Pistoia," *Economic History Review*, 2d ser., 18 (1965), pp. 225–44.

24. Michael Dols, *The Black Death in the Middle East* (Princeton, N.J., 1977).

25. Lawrence Langer, "Plague and the Russian Countryside: Monastic Estates in the Late Fourteenth and Fifteenth Centuries," *Canadian-American Slavic Studies* 10 (1976):351–68.

26. Robert S. Gottfried, *Epidemic Disease in Fifteenth-Century England: The Medical Response and the Demographic Consequences* (New Brunswick, N.J., 1978). A review by Joseph Shatzmiller appears in *Speculum* 54 (1979):378–79.

27. See, for example, the article by Bowsky cited in n. 23 above, and Richard W. Emery, "The Black Death of 1348 in Perpignan," *Speculum*

42 (1967):611–23; Susan M. Stuard, "Public Health: Social Cohesion and Quarantine, Rational Responses to Plague in Medieval Ragusa," presented at the CEMERS Conference, may also be cited in this connection. For the response in Florence, see n. 7 to the essay by Aldo Bernardo, below, p. 62.

28. See Michael Dols, "The Second Plague Pandemic and Its Recurrences in the Middle East, 1347–1894," *Journal of the Economic and Social History of the Orient* 23 (Paris, 1979), pp. 162–89.

29. By Manfred Ullmann, *Die Medizin im Islam* (Leiden-Köln, 1970), and Fuat Sezgin, *Geschichte der arabischen Schrifttums*, 6 vols. (Leiden, 1967–78), 3: "Medizin – Pharmazie – Zoologie – Tierheilkunde bis ca. 430 H" (1970).

The Black Death: The Crisis
and Its Social
and Economic Consequences .

J. M. W. Bean

The removal of cataclysms is almost an occupational disease of modern historians because a critical approach to contemporary evidence leads quite naturally to suspicion of contemporary stress on the consequences of great events or of the work of professional colleagues whose reputations are based on the discovery of crises. The Black Death in Western Europe has not escaped such attempts to scale it down. Nevertheless it has survived, on the whole, remarkably well as one of the great events and turning points in European history since the fall of Rome. The explanation lies partly in the horror and helplessness which find full expression in the chronicles of the Black Death, but it can also be found in the very nature of our evidence. The search for statistics relating to actual death rates is a comparatively recent development; and what details have so far been discovered are sporadic in their chronological and geographical coverage. Moreover, even when sources yielding such data have all been found and completely exhausted, the same limitations are still bound to apply. In consequence, the historian of the Black Death can never escape completely from the details and patterns imposed by the chronicles' accounts.

Over the past twenty-five years, however, we have been in a much better position to evaluate both the chronicles and the statistical evidence. In the plague pandemic which ravaged the Far East and India from 1894 onwards medical authorities were confronted with plague as an opponent in the hospital ward, not merely as a story of the ineffectiveness and superstition of their predecessors from the fourteenth through the eighteenth centuries. With the publication of the general treatises by Hirst[1] and Pollitzer[2] medical research on plague became easily available and comprehensible to historians. Its conclusions have certainly been mirrored in recent historical work — for example, in the study of the Black Death in Orvieto by Carpentier[3] and in her more general sketch,[4] or in the general popular account by Ziegler.[5] Even so, insufficient effort has been given to the analysis of the chronicle sources and existing statistical evidence in the light of modern medical knowledge.[6] What this paper will try to do is to show how a critical use of modern medical knowledge can illuminate our understanding of the spread of plague in the years 1347–1350 and show how this can assist the social and the economic historian in assessing the severity of the consequent loss of life.

In the closing paper of this conference it may be unnecessary to summarize modern medical knowledge. But some reminders are essential for what is to follow. Modern medicine knows three types of plague, caused fundamentally by the same bacillus — bubonic, pneumonic, and septicaemic. The septicaemic type can be dismissed from our calculations at the start. It is extremely virulent and explains the stories we occasionally encounter of plague victims suddenly dropping dead. When this occurred, infestation with plague bacilli was so enormous that there was no time for other symptoms to appear. Septicaemic infection was thus a special by-product of other types of plague. The most well-known form is the bubonic, so called because of its visible symptoms, the buboes that most frequently appear in the groin or armpits, the region of major lymphatic glands which the plague bacillus attacks. Pneumonic plague remains something of a mystery in its origins. The most likely explanation for its appearance lies in plague infection of victims who were at the same time suffering from pneumonia. A mutation then occurred, producing a disease with the symptoms of a violent and deadly pneumonia. For the historian there are vital differences between the bubonic and pneumonic types of plague. First, the bubonic form is in a special sense contagious, being caused by the bite of a flea that has fled from a dead, or dying, rat victim, while the pneumonic strain can be spread by droplets of moisture coughed or spat out by victims. Pneumonic plague thus spreads much more easily. Second, the rat flea which usually spreads the bubonic form propagates most abundantly in a damp climate with a temperature ranging between 68° and 78° Fahrenheit. But the association of the pneumonic form with pneumonia means that in Western Europe it was bound to be a disease primarily of the winter months. Third, pneumonic plague is a virtually fatal disease, probably the speediest and deadliest killer known to man, whereas recovery from the bubonic variety is possible.

This account, however, does not exhaust the details about plague required by historians. The most important key to the understanding of the disease is a simple fact: it is primarily a disease of rats, not human beings. Bubonic plague, and pneumonic in the first instance, are transmitted to man only when its fleas leave the dead or dying rat victim and find a temporary home on a human host. The rat population and its fleas form a permanent reservoir of plague. Human beings are only at risk when climatic conditions encourage the breeding of the fleas. The rat of the Middle Ages — the black rat — invariably lived close to, or in, human habitations.

As far as we know, when plague came from the East via the Black Sea in 1347, the rat population of Western Europe did not harbor plague. It had to be infected before humans were. Moreover, because the black rat invariably dwelt close to, or even in, human habitations, there were considerable limits to the speed with which plague could travel. Present scientific knowledge compels us to dismiss any notion that plague travelled from one center of human population to another, using the rats of the intervening countryside as a sort of bridge. Instead, what happened was that rats bearing their fleas travelled in ships. Alternatively, the vermin could travel over land with their favorite food, grain; or the fleas alone (which can survive days away from their hosts) went in bales of merchandise, most probably cloth or wool.

Much of this information has already had some effect on recent accounts of the Black Death in Europe. The role of pneumonic plague was, for example, stressed years ago by Carpentier in both her study of Orvieto and in her general article. Above all, there is now common agreement that the nature of plague and the behavior of its hosts explain the directions it took once it had arrived in the Western Mediterranean in 1347. It first attacked the ports of Messina, Genoa and Venice, and then traveled to Marseilles and from there up the Rhone. It did not reach Paris until the summer of 1348. And the same summer saw its arrival on the south coast of England. Perhaps the most striking evidence of the dependence of plague on the trade routes is to be found outside Western Europe, in the fact that Novgorod received it from Baltic trade, rather than directly from its original home in Central Asia.

But at this point we must part company with the previous accounts and press further into this basic chronological framework. Contemporary descriptions support the view of Hirst and others that the Black Death comprised pneumonic as well as bubonic elements. The most clinical study is Guy de Chaulliac's description of victims' symptoms at Avignon. References to the spitting of blood by the afflicted can be found in the chronicles' description of the epidemics of Messina, Venice and other Italian cities, and at Almeira in Spain. And its presence in the British Isles may be inferred from a similar reference in Ireland. These accounts apart, can the absence of a pneumonic element be assumed if there is no contemporary reference to its symptoms? At this point medical knowledge comes to our aid: it is reasonable to assume that, if an outbreak raged through the winter, there was pneumonic plague. And, of course, we know that our most detailed description of pneumonic symptoms came from an account composed during a winter outbreak. Does this conclusion, however, mean that a summer outbreak meant the absence of pneumonic plague? On this point the conclusions of Carpentier about Orvieto imply a negative answer. In her description of its plague she describes how the disease raged there through the summer of 1348 and argues for a pneumonic as well as bubonic outbreak on the basis of a source describing the plague in Florence.[7] Her interpretation should, I believe, be treated with scepticism. A distinction must be made between epidemic pneumonic plague and the individual cases of this form that, in the absence of the necessary climatic conditions, could not start an epidemic. Nor can we exclude the possibility that especially virulent infections by plague bacilli had led to a spitting or vomiting of blood which was caused by hemorrhage of the lungs.[8] At any rate, it is difficult to believe that a pneumonic element was more than a secondary factor in the death rate at Orvieto. And the arguments on which this conclusion is based have implications beyond the history of this single city. The outbreaks in the inland cities of Tuscany (recent scholarship[9] has examined Siena[10] and Pistoia[11]) were all summer outbreaks.

What emerges from this discussion is a rough pattern of plague outbreaks in Western Europe in 1347–49. Winter outbreaks occurred in Provence, centering on Avignon; in Paris and parts of northern France, including Normandy; and in parts of England. All these visitations must have been primarily epidemics of pneumonic plague. In contrast, we must assume that inland Tuscany had primarily bubonic epidemics. In France a few cities in the south have been studied;[12] there also the outbreaks took place in summer and were hence, presumably, bubonic. From this rough pattern we may proceed to argue that the death rates in England, in parts of northern France and in Provence must have been markedly higher than in inland Tuscany. There is, however, one obvious body of information in the way of this theory. Recent researches on the death rates in Tuscany and central Italy suggest that the percentage of fatalities in this area was very high — fifty percent in Orvieto[13] and Siena,[14] and fifty-eight percent in San Gimignano.[15] But these estimates need not present so powerful an obstacle as they appear at first sight to offer. In the first place, these statistics, whether chroniclers' or modern historians', all refer to cities. We should not assume that the same estimates should be applied to the surrounding countryside. And the mechanics of plague transmission give support to this counter-argument. The route of travel followed by the chief agent — the grain trade — led out of the *contado*, not into it. In the second place, the account of the coming of plague which is probably the most famous of all — the opening of the *Decameron* of Boccaccio — tells how his storytellers fled into the countryside to escape the afflictions of the city.

This pattern of the uneven incidence of the destruction of human life by plague in Western Europe will deservedly invite scepticism because it erects theory on interpretation. And, when one moves away from France, Italy and England, one enters countries that have received much less attention from this standpoint. Details, for example, of severe death rates are available for some Hanseatic cities,[16] but the archives of other areas of Germany, especially those of the cities of the Rhineland, still await investigation. Even so, it is also worth looking at the other side of the coin. This consists of those areas which suffered very little, if at all, from the Black Death. The extent to which this can be said with confidence of large areas of Eastern Europe is uncertain, because present knowledge is fragmentary and confused. There is, however, apparent unanimity of scholarly opinion that, apart from Flanders, the Low Countries largely escaped and that Bohemia was untouched. Explanations are available for these phenomena. In the case of Bohemia there is the chronicler's statement that, when the plague arrived at its borders, the climate was too cold for it to proceed further. In the case of the Low Countries there is the modern suggestion that fishing and stock farming gave the inhabitants plenty of protein.[17] But the mechanics of the spread of plague provide a more acceptable interpretation. Plague could only arrive in Bohemia by travelling overland; and this was also one of the two kinds of routes by which it approached the Low Countries — eastwards from nor-

thern France and northwards from the Rhineland. But these routes
began in areas of virulent outbreaks among the human populations; and the severity of the visitations imply in turn an equally
violent devastation of the rat population. The most reasonable
hypothesis is that the destruction of the rat population destroyed
the source from which the plague-bearing fleas could renew their
supplies of plague bacilli, while the disruption of trade caused by
the extreme violence of the human outbreak meant that few of the
infected parasites left the region. For plague-free areas of the Low
Countries, to be sure, we must look for an additional explanation
that will account for the failure of the disease to arrive in epidemic
proportions in the North Sea ports. But shipping that brought
plague-bearing rats and fleas had to come from England or from
the south via the Channel — in other words, from areas so badly
disrupted that few ships could have sailed from them.

None of these arguments underrates the crisis as a whole. Rather,
they serve collectively to suggest that a comparison between regions,
produced by the study of contemporary evidence in the light of
modern medical knowledge, is a beneficial approach to a study of
the social and economic consequences of the Black Death. In a
paper[18] published in 1963 I argued that a distinction should be
drawn in the case of England between the Black Death and the
plague epidemics which followed that apocalyptic affliction. Here,
however, I am arguing that the Black Death should not be regarded as a unitary force. The truth is that historians' discussions of
the economic effects of the Black Death fall into two categories:
local studies of death rates on the one hand, and, on the other,
wide-ranging interpretations which speak of a global death rate and
seek to place the crisis in the setting of a declining European
economy over a period of one and a half centuries.

Attempts at synthesis are essential, true, but there is no justification for the faith so often placed in blanket theories when there
are so many areas of ignorance. If we are to engage in some tentative generalizations while at the same time we proceed in the investigation of the archives, it is best to do so within the framework
of regional comparisons. And it can also be argued that the
generalizations offered by the present paper have interesting implications. If inland Tuscany suffered marginally less from the Black
Death than other areas of Western Europe, does not this fact offer
us some insight into its economic situation in the late fourteenth
and fifteenth centuries? According to some authorities Milan suf-

fered less than other Italian cities. Does this statement help us to understand Milanese power under the last Visconti and the Sforzas? Does Bohemia's exemption from the ravages of the Black Death help to explain its comparative prosperity in the reign of Charles IV of Luxemburg? Similarly, the comparative immunity of the hinterland of Antwerp must have provided a labour supply which assisted that area's economic growth over the next century and a half.

The loose and hypothetical character of these remarks is in some measure due to two difficulties. One is the comparative lack of evidence, a condition which may well subsist when all the archives have been thoroughly searched. The other is the tendency for that evidence to be urban in provenance. Neither of these difficulties, however, is encountered in one area of Western Europe — England. During this period that country was free from one influence which had economic consequences that are difficult to disentangle from those of the Black Death itself: the devastation of war, which, for example, makes the analysis of the northern French situation so difficult. For these reasons it may be useful to close with some comments on England. The Black Death there has been studied from two angles. One is the incidence of death rates, the latest contribution being the first chapters of the book by Shrewsbury.[19] The other is the statistics unearthed by the economic historian. Some comments on Shrewsbury's work are in order because it has the appearance of majesty and learning which gives force to its author's conclusion that the Black Death carried off a mere one-twentieth of the population. Shrewsbury simply states that pneumonic plague cannot exist independently of a bubonic outbreak. He thus dismisses as evidence of plague the materials that reveal a winter epidemic. Similarly, his view that the Black Death did not affect the nobility and gentry can easily be disproved: the evidence of inquisitions *post mortem*, which relate to the upper landed classes, indicates that the death rate was roughly ten times the normal one in the year or so following the advent of the Black Death (though mainly, it must be said, in the summer of 1349).[20]

Shrewsbury's errors arise from his determination to downplay the role of plague as distinct from other epidemic diseases in the England of 1348-49. Once we discard some of Shrewsbury's premises we are forced to dismiss additionally his view that the plague was a mainly urban phenomenon. The details he provides show, in fact, that it reached country areas — for example, the borders of Wales, a predominantly pastoral area. At the same time

his compilation of available statistics also reveals considerable variations in the local death rates, which range from one-fifth to two-
thirds within the ranks of the manorial tenantry. What emerges
from Shrewsbury's compilation of detail, shorn of its author's
preconceptions and *idées fixes*, is the conclusion that the spread of
plague within England presents the same pattern as we see in
Western Europe as a whole, spreading slowly from the ports inland. England appears as a microcosm demonstrating within its
boundaries the regional and local variations in incidence of infection that can be seen on a larger scale in Western Europe as a whole.

This is a picture that agrees well with the work of economic
historians on the manorial evidence. Decades ago Professor Levett
showed that a sample of the manors of the Bishop of Winchester
weathered the Black Death.[21] Vacant holdings were soon taken up;
and the Bishop's loss of rents was more than compensated for
through entry fines and heriots. More recently, the same picture
has emerged from the study of other manors, notably some in East
Anglia.[22] But the very same volume as contained Professor Levett's
study also contained details of other Winchester manors whose
holdings remained vacant for decades and experienced a severe loss
of revenues,[23] a point which Professor Postan strengthened and
developed in 1949.[24]

The merit of some discussion of England is that it pinpoints the
difficulties inherent in any attempt to relate the loss of life through
the Black Death to the development of the economy as a whole.
Some years ago A. R. Bridbury[25] sought to play down the Black
Death's importance in itself, arguing that "if it is ever to be restored
to favour as a dynamic force in fourteenth-century history, then
it is in the seventies, rather than in the mid-century decades that
it has dominated for so long, that the Black Death must be found
a tenable position to occupy." Substantial difficulties are presented
by this statement. Indeed, its rhetoric seems to arrogate to the
historian the authority to move a known event from its actual place
in time. It appears to mean that the crisis in the fortunes of landowners and their tenants was not really felt until the fourteen-
seventies. It is certainly possible to deal with Bridbury's comments
on our lack of knowledge concerning the plagues that occurred in
the quarter-century following the Black Death. If we regard the
statistics of the inquisitions *post mortem* as a sort of barometer of
the severity of the respective plagues, we do not find it easy to believe
that those of 1369 and 1375 depressed the population level further.[26]

To be sure, the death rate of 1361 was seven times the normal, as compared with the Black Death's ten. But this should not be interpreted as an indication that the plague of 1361 produced deaths to a level not remarkably below that of the Black Death: plague, when it arrived in human habitations, struck first among the poor and took a long time (as in 1348–49 itself) to reach the upper ranks of landed society. The comparable figures for 1369 and 1375 are roughly three times the average. If we take into account the usual tendency of the birth rate to rise after a devastating epidemic, we can certainly allow the plague of 1361 an importance that we must deny to those of 1369 and 1375.

This point apart, the arguments presented by Bridbury are basically twofold—first, the fact that wage rates did not soar to the level we might expect if the death rate were as high as one-third or so; and, second, the evidence that on some estates revenues remained buoyant until the last three-quarters of the century. It is tempting to dismiss these arguments by the easiest and most readily available means—the limited character of the evidence accessible. Evidence of prices and wages come essentially from two sources—the Oxford and Cambridge college archives searched by Thordd Rogers and the estates of the Bishops of Winchester, together with the more interpretive statistics of real wages calculated by the Phelps Brown-Hopkins index. Similarly, scarcely a handful of landed estates have received anything approaching the treatment they would require to give an adequate foundation to Bridbury's generalizations.

But it is necessary to go deeper. Bridbury's approach presents us with a conception of the untrammelled operation of market forces that is alien to the agrarian economy of the Middle Ages. Most of the agrarian products of the era of the Black Death came from the peasant farmer, not the great landowner, a fact which historians forget in their obsession with demesne-farming by the lord. When great landowners like the Bishops of Winchester paid wages to agricultural laborers, they were doing so to peasants many, if not most, of whom were their villeins and for this reason less able to bargain freely. Even so, there was a pronounced rise in wages. And we should beware of arguing that the real value of wages in the decade following the Black Death was reduced by a series of bad harvests. Are we to believe that most peasants bought their corn on the market? A bad harvest meant that they had less to sell. It is also a fact that eighty years before the Black Death the Hundred Rolls revealed in the Midlands a peasantry of which twenty-nine percent possessed holdings insufficient to maintain themselves and their families. It can be argued that these must have suffered more than other peasants from the great famine of 1315–17. On the other hand, most of them, the cottars, lived on the edges of manors and may have been marginally less liable to the ravages of plague than those who lived in the center of the settlement. Their existence has long been accepted as the reason why holdings were taken up quickly in many manors in the aftermath of the Black Death. Equally, on some estates (and those of the Bishop of Winchester must be numbered among them) their presence constituted a brake on the use of agricultural wages.

There are two especially serious objections to Bridbury's arguments. His view of the working of the manor is rather unsophisticated. Part of the lord's revenues came from a body of rents fixed by custom: if the original tenant's family continued in the direct line, the rent of a holding could remain fixed for centuries. The deaths of tenants without heirs during the Black Death enabled lords to demand market rents, an important element in the tendency of the revenues of some manors to remain stable. Buoyancy of landowners' incomes, therefore, is not a satisfactory argument against the view that the Black Death removed a substantial portion of the population. Nor can an analysis that deals with arable farming by lords and peasants and with grain prices give a complete account of the agrarian economy. Many peasants were sheep owners; indeed, the greater part of England's wool production was always in their hands. Sheep did not suffer from plague. And the fifteen years from 1353 onwards were boom years for English cloth exports. In short, there is not convincing evidence that the Black Death in England was not a serious crisis. In particular, an estimate of a total death rate of thirty percent or so has yet to be disproved.

An examination of the case of England along these lines is a useful way of bringing this discussion to an end because it brings home the extent to which any study of the economic consequences of the Black Death must always remain open-ended. Contemporary comment we have to distrust; outside a few sources such as English bishops' registers, the evidence of death rates is local and for most settlements we have no information. And, if we argue from economic evidence, we deal with data that may mirror other factors. These limitations apply equally to continental Europe; and they will still be present when all the archives have been investigated. It is the historian's task to search for patterns in the events and phenomena he studies. It is the thesis of this paper that patterns in the impact of the Black Death can only be traced if we pay careful attention to medical knowledge. What we already know permits us to observe marked regional variations in the severity of the death rate.

The role of these regional variations in the economic development of continental Europe deserves more attention. Indeed, in some of these regions we can go further along the road of tentative generalization, due to the existence in continental Europe of large urban centers. Because of this, in Germany, Lombardy, and Tuscany a powerful element in the shock given to the economy by the Black Death must be found in the devastation it wrought in the urban markets for agricultural produce.

It is in regional and intra-regional comparisons of this sort that we must seek to evaluate the economic consequences of the Black Death. Distrust of contemporary comment cannot negate the actual fact of an enormous loss of life. Attempts to downplay the importance of the Black Death, whether on a national scale like those of Shrewsbury and Bridbury or a more local scale like that of Levett, are misconceived. The most fruitful line of investigation lies in regional and intra-regional comparisons. The lesson of the present state of scholarship concerning the consequences of the Black Death is that it was a powerful but blunt instrument which left uneven injuries.

J. M. W. Bean

Deaths Recorded in Inquisitions Post Mortem, 1344–1375

(M = Males   F = Females   T = Total)

		Jan-Feb	Mar-Apr	May-June	July-Aug	Sept-Oct	Nov-Dec	Total
1344	M	7	5	3	2	9	6	32
	F	4	2	3	—	2	3	14
	T	11	7	6	2	11	9	46
1345	M	9	6	2	6	4	7	34
	F	1	1	2	2	2	2	10
	T	10	7	4	8	6	9	44
1346	M	5	6	5	7	8	10	41
	F	4	—	2	3	2	—	11
	T	9	6	7	10	10	10	52
1347	M	6	5	5	8	10	12	46
	F	3	1	1	4	—	1	10
	T	9	6	6	12	10	13	56
1348	M	3	10	4	4	11	9	41
	F	5	11	7	6	17	11	57
	T	8	21	11	10	28	20	98
1349	M	12	33	80	141	58	15	339
	F	3	13	22	39	20	1	98
	T	15	46	102	180	78	16	437
1350	M	3	6	6	10	6	2	33
	F	1	2	1	4	4	—	12
	T	4	8	7	14	10	2	45
1351	M	6	4	8	4	5	1	28
	F	—	—	1	—	—	1	2
	T	6	4	9	4	5	2	30
1352	M	6	5	5	5	9	6	36
	F	1	—	1	1	—	1	4
	T	7	5	6	6	9	7	40
1353	M	3	5	6	5	7	7	33
	F	1	2	1	1	—	3	8
	T	4	7	7	6	7	10	41

1354	M	3	4	5	6	7	3	28
	F	2	5	—	3	—	2	12
	T	5	9	5	9	7	5	40
1355	M	3	5	3	4	7	3	25
	F	2	2	1	1	—	—	6
	T	5	7	4	5	7	3	31
1356	M	3	3	6	3	6	2	23
	F	2	—	2	1	2	1	8
	T	5	3	8	4	8	3	31
1357	M	4	3	3	5	3	1	19
	F	—	1	2	1	—	2	6
	T	4	4	5	6	3	3	25
1358	M	4	6	4	5	3	5	27
	F	—	1	—	1	4	2	8
	T	4	7	4	6	7	7	35
1359	M	5	3	8	2	8	6	32
	F	1	1	4	1	—	1	8
	T	6	4	12	3	8	7	40
1360	M	9	7	7	12	11	7	53
	F	—	2	4	1	—	2	9
	T	9	9	11	13	11	9	62
1361	M	4	8	20	59	112	54	257
	F	2	—	4	21	36	18	81
	T	6	8	24	80	148	72	338
1362	M	18	8	11	9	12	2	60
	F	2	5	4	2	4	3	20
	T	20	13	15	11	16	5	80
1363	M	2	2	3	6	8	3	24
	F	—	—	4	1	3	2	10
	T	2	2	7	7	11	5	34
1364	M	6	3	4	3	6	2	24
	F	—	—	1	3	—	—	4
	T	6	3	5	6	6	2	28
1365	M	2	1	8	4	3	4	22
	F	—	1	2	1	2	2	8
	T	2	2	10	5	5	6	30

1366	M	3	6	3	1	3	5	21
	F	1	1	2	–	1	–	5
	T	4	7	5	1	4	5	26
1367	M	4	10	2	11	4	3	34
	F	2	1	2	2	–	1	8
	T	6	11	4	13	4	4	40
1368	M	6	2	7	8	9	6	38
	F	–	4	–	2	3	3	12
	T	6	6	7	10	12	9	50
1369	M	6	2	12	40	39	11	110
	F	–	–	2	17	14	5	38
	T	6	2	14	57	53	16	148
1370	M	3	1	5	9	4	7	29
	F	–	2	–	1	–	–	3
	T	3	3	5	10	4	7	32
1371	M	3	1	3	1	10	6	24
	F	1	4	–	2	–	–	7
	T	4	5	3	3	10	6	31
1372	M	3	6	5	6	4	5	29
	F	1	2	1	1	1	5	11
	T	4	8	6	7	5	10	40
1373	M	3	5	6	1	3	4	22
	F	1	–	–	3	3	2	9
	T	4	5	6	4	6	6	31
1374	M	4	8	2	4	6	3	27
	F	–	2	1	–	5	1	9
	T	4	10	3	4	11	4	36
1375	M	5	8	12	19	31	11	86
	F	2	1	3	11	15	6	38
	T	7	9	15	30	46	17	124

notes

1. L. Fabian Hirst, *The Conquest of Plague: A Study of the Evolution of Epidemiology* (Oxford, 1953).

2. R. Pollitzer, *Plague*, World Health Organization, Monograph Series, no. 22 (Geneva, 1954).

3. Elisabeth Carpentier, *Une ville devant la Peste: Orvieto et la Peste Noire de 1348* (Paris, 1952).

4. Elisabeth Carpentier, "Autour de la Peste Noire: Famines et épidémies dans l'histoire du XIVe siècle," *Annales: Economies, Sociétés, Civilisations* 17 (1962):1062-92.

5. Philip Ziegler, *The Black Death* (New York, 1969).

6. The best detailed summary of the chronicle evidence remains that of Francis A. Gasquet, *The Black Death of 1348 and 1349* (London, 1908), originally published as *The Great Pestilence* (London, 1893).

7. Carpentier, *Une ville*, pp. 99-101.

8. Bubonic plague often creates lung lesions.

9. Contemporary accounts indicate that the outbreak in Florence was also in the summer.

10. W. M. Bowsky, "The Impact of the Black Death upon Sienese Government and Society," *Speculum* 39 (1964):1-34.

11. David Herlihy, *Medieval and Renaissance Pistoia* (New Haven, Conn., 1967).

12. For example, see G. Prat, "Albi et la Peste Noire," *Annales du Midi* 64 (1952); P. Wolff, "Trois études de démographie mediévale en France méridionale," *Studi in onore d'Armando Sapori*, 2 vols. (Milan, 1957); R. W. Emery, "The Black Death of 1348 in Perpignan," *Speculum* 42 (1967): 611-23.

13. Carpentier, *Une ville*, p. 135.

14. Bowsky, art. cit., p. 18.

15. E. Fiumi, "La popolazione. . . . volterrano-sangimignanese," *Studi in onore di Amintore Fanfani* (Milan, 1962), p. 280.

16. Cited in Carpentier, art. cit., p. 1065, nn. 2-3.

17. For example, see B. H. Slicher Van Bath, *The Agrarian History of Western Europe, A.D. 500-1850* (London, 1965), p. 89.

18. "Plague, Population and Economic Decline in England in the Later Middle Ages," *Economic History Review*, 2 Ser. 15 (1962-1963): 423-37.

19. J. F. D. Shrewsbury, *A History of the Bubonic Plague in the British Isles* (Cambridge, England, 1970).

20. See Appendix. This summarizes the dates of death supplied in the printed *Calendar of Inquisitions Post Mortem*. The breakdown into bi-monthly periods makes it possible to estimate the presence of pneumonic plague in the winter and also to check whether plague was present outside the years 1348-49, 1361, 1369 and 1375.

21. In volume 5 (1916) of P. Vinogradoff, ed., *Oxford Studies in Social and Legal History.*

22. *G. A. Holmes, The Estates of the Higher Nobility in Fourteenth-Century England* (Cambridge, 1957), p. 114.

23. The chapter by A. Ballard.

24. M. Postan, "Some Economic Evidence of Declining Population in the Later Middle Ages," *Economic History Review*, 2d ser. 2 (1949–50), pp. 221–89, especially 241–42.

25. A. R. Bridbury, "The Black Death," *Economic History Review*, 2d ser. 26 (1973), pp. 557–92.

26. See Appendix.

the plague as key to meaning in Boccaccio's "Decameron"

Aldo S. Bernardo

hardly anyone can dispute the importance of those sections of Boccaccio's *Decameron* in which the author addresses the reader, just as no one can doubt the central importance of the so-called frame story in defining the basic structure of Boccaccio's masterpiece. Yet, while admitting such importance few critics have done more than consider these portions embarrassing but necessary intrusions that constitute one of the work's imperfections. The stories, for such critics, are all that really matter. The various components of the framework are mere devices for getting the stories under way or for justifying their nature and value.

Recent criticism, however, has begun to reexamine the work as a whole and has begun to detect within it new dimensions of meaning. Accepting the masterfully artistic nature of the individual stories, these critics have turned to the problem of unity of the whole, and have begun to attack on an understandably broad basis those elements which have led Robert Hollander to observe, "The work remains . . . possibly the most enigmatic text in continental medieval fiction, richly difficult to fathom."[1]

The purpose of this paper is to analyze in some detail the four sections that constitute the frame or superstructure of the tales in order to show the extent to which these sections (especially the Introduction with its description of the plague) contribute to the meaning of the whole by providing signs or signals intended to guide the alert reader. In this manner I hope to establish certain lines of development which would afford the reader at least a balanced perspective from which to approach the tales as a unified whole, one that would go beyond the bounds of naturalism which lately have been wanting found as the basis of the work's form.

The frame of the work consists of three sections in which the author/narrator addresses the reader directly, and one section, the frame *story*, which speaks of the *brigata* of ten young people who become the narrators of the tales. Boccaccio, as the narrator/author, addresses the reader three times at considerable length — in the *Proem*, in the *Introduction to Day IV* and finally in the *Conclusion*. The frame story's keystone is the *Introduction* in which it is set in motion, while its evolving form recurs regularly, primarily at the beginning and end of each day and of each story. That the author intended these sections of his work to be just as integral a part of the whole as the 100 tales is perfectly clear.

Before turning to the *Proem* proper we must note an important particular. Since the manuscript tradition of the *Decameron* shows the title to be an integral part of the *Proem* (as well as part of the *explicit*), it is essential that we begin with the full title: "Here begins the book called *Decameron*, otherwise known as Prince Galahalt, wherein are contained a hundred stories, told in ten days by seven ladies and three young men."[2] Anyone familiar with the canto of Paola and Francesca in Dante's *Inferno* will recognize the inference immediately. The sin and subsequent punishment visited upon Dante's two lovers resulted from an illicit passion which overwhelmed the lovers as they read from a book containing the tale of the sweet loves of Lancelot and Guinevere. According to Dante the book had served as a Prince Galehaut, the famed courtly pander who had arranged the secret meetings of the two lovers. It was therefore an instrument of death for Dante's two lovers notwithstanding its popularity as a courtly romance. Consequently one can only conclude from Boccaccio's subtitle that his book, too, may be an instrument of death and destruction if not read with care.[3]

If we now examine the *Proem*, the very first sentence, despite its famous first two words, "Umana cosa," establishes a clearly Augustinian mood: "To take pity on people in distress is a human quality. . . ."[4] Charity toward one's fellow man is what one must observe, especially if one has been helped by the charity of others to overcome a dangerous affliction which ought to be shunned. The affliction itself is Augustinian: love as an overwhelming passion. And Augustinian is the remedy: learn to withstand passion, for time will eventually snuff it out.

The love from which the narrator had been freed had indeed been "altissimo" and "nobile", but ill-regulated appetite had caused this love to become "a craving that was ill-restrained." Thanks to understanding and sympathetic friends who tried to console him through endless, though seemingly fruitless, conversations, he avoided certain death. God, however, through His grace brought an end to the overwhelming passion just as He is wont to do with all things in this life. What remained of the passion was a pleasurable feeling deriving from the awareness of having escaped a destructive force.

The narrator then points out that though his suffering is gone there still remains the recollection of the role played by friends in liberating him. Since he considers gratitude among the greatest virtues he now hopes to do for others in his former condition what his friends had done for him. Fortunately his friends, either through wisdom or good fortune, did not themselves need such assistance. He therefore proposes to direct his assistance to those who have the greatest need: fair ladies in love who suffer the flames of love in a most unfortunate manner — alone and in their rooms — unlike men who can participate in activities that help keep their minds occupied and hence free from the excesses of love. His plan is to offer what he calls "nuovi ragionamenti" that may help them dispel the melancholia they suffer. Therefore in order to remedy this unfair female inferiority perpetrated by Fortune he will tell a hundred stories for their pleasure as told by seven ladies and three men, during the recent plague, according to an unspecified informant, as well as some of the songs they sang for their own pleasure. Good and bad love will be the main subject as well as other topics that had been of interest in both ancient and modern times. These stories will be not only a source of enjoyment, but a source of useful advice. In them will be shown what is to be avoided and what is to be pursued. This knowledge will help the young ladies overcome their affliction. But the book is the real message; the tales are only the means; the ladies in love are to focus their attention on what the book as a whole is saying.

In a recent article Branca shows in great detail the similarity between Boccaccio's *Proem* and the first sonnet of Petrarch's *Canzoniere*, thereby establishing recantation as the basic motif of the *Proem*.[5] The theme of having escaped a fate similar to death through the grace of God echoes St. Augustine's truancy as described in his *Confessions*. In Petrarch's *Secretum* Augustinus gives Franciscus precisely the advice implicit in the *Proem*. The obvious Dantean note of the subtitle recalls both the *Vita nuova* and the *Divine Com-*

edy, and reminds the fair ladies in love not to fall into the same
trap as did Dante's two famous lovers. The work is obviously meant
to help others avoid the temptations of carnal love, but it must be
read with care, for the author's attempt to make it interesting may
contain the seed of perdition as did that other book about illicit
love for Dante's two unalert readers. Boccaccio's *Proem* thus contains Augustinian, Petrarchan and Dantean echoes.

   Just as the subtitle is part of the *Proem* so is the *Introduction*, describing the plague, part of the first day. As such it is integral to the
main body of the work. Since it literally opens the work it must
be considered, according to medieval literary aesthetics, extremely significant. It starts with a passage that recalls the initial moments
of Dante's *Comedy*. Upon returning from his unique journey Dante
felt moved to open his account with some horrendous details
necessary to a full understanding of his experience, "But to reveal
the good that I found there/ I will speak first of other things."[6] Boccaccio also is aware that the opening of his work will likewise appear "irksome and ponderous" to his "fairest ladies," but, like Dante,
he reassures them that this does not mean that their journey will
be in "an endless torrent of tears and sobbing." His grim beginning will likewise be like climbing "a steep and rugged hill," but
the more difficult the climb the more delightful will be the plain
that will eventually be reached, echoing Proverbs 14:13. Like Dante,
Boccaccio would have preferred to avoid such a shocking beginning, but in order to achieve his desired end he too felt moved to
include such an account. Indeed, as he arrives at the end of his
justification, he repeats, "I really have no alternative but to address
myself to its composition," recalling *Inferno* xxxii,6, "not without
fear do I bring myself to speak." Indeed, if one listens closely, echoes
of Petrarch's climb of Mt. Ventoux may likewise be heard.

   There follows the account of the plague whose opening contrasts
the life-giving Incarnation of Christ and the superior beauty of
Florence with the "mortifera pestilenza" which is clearly associated
with divine wrath rather than planetary influences since it arrived
from the East and assumed different symptoms in the West. The
apocalyptic ring of the opening is unmistakable: "The deadly
pestilence . . . through the influence of the heavenly bodies [or as]
a punishment signifying God's righteous anger at our iniquitous
way of life . . . originated some years earlier in the East, where
it had claimed countless lives before it unhappily spread westward,
growing in strength as it swept relentlessly on from one place to
the next."[7]

The relentless progress of the affliction and its inevitable fatality are contrasted with specific behavior patterns of the Florentines, patterns which, like the plague itself, followed no logical form. The extremes of conduct consisted on the one hand of moderation in consuming the very finest foods in isolation and on the other of living life to the fullest in various homes where only the most pleasant and entertaining subjects were discussed. The mean, ironically, consisted in satisfying one's appetite to the extreme, wandering wherever one pleased. The safest alternative was to run away and abandon the incredible scenes of human suffering and of man's inhumanity to man, especially as exemplified in the actions of blood relatives. "It was not merely a question of one citizen avoiding another, and of people almost invariably neglecting their neighbors and rarely or never visiting their relatives, addressing them only from a distance. . . ."[8] What was worse was that ". . . brothers abandoned brothers, uncles their nephews, sisters their brothers, and in many cases wives deserted their husbands. But even worse, and almost incredible, was the fact that fathers and mothers refused to nurse and assist their own children as though they did not belong to them."[9] The description reaches a climax with the astonishing statistic that "between March and July of the year in question . . . it is reliably thought that over a hundred thousand human lives were extinguished within the walls of the city of Florence. Yet before this lethal catastrophe fell upon the city, it is doubtful whether anyone would have guessed it contained so many inhabitants."[10] By the time the description is concluded one senses that it indeed parallels the mad activities of Dante's *Inferno*, with the Florentines obviously indulging in acts of incontinence, violence, and fraud. The basic bestiality of the populace clearly reminds one of the evil love of self, while the terrible contagion that struck down even swine is reminiscent of the contagiousness of such love, recalling by association the wicked passion of Paolo and Francesca. As in the *Comedy* the imagery of animality becomes intensified as the description draws to a close.[11]

As the focus turns to the account of the meeting of the *brigata* there is an almost dazzling display of numerology to indicate the extent to which God's hand seems to be everywhere and yet unrecognized. First there is the very year of the plague itself, 1348, whose outer numbers add up to 9 and inner ones to 7. Then there are the 7 ladies whose number is enlarged to 10 by 3 men. The oldest lady is 27 (a nine), the youngest 18 (a nine). The difference

between the two ages is 9. If these two ages are subtracted from
1348 the totals are respectively 1321 (a 7) and 1330 (another 7).
The minimum age of the men (25) also totals 7, while the names
of the ladies are given in two groups of 4 and 3, and we first see
them sitting in a circle composed of 3 on one side, 3 on another
and 1 in the center. [12] It is possible of course that, in keeping with
the mercantile humor that had begun to permeate his works following his return to Florence, Boccaccio is here "having fun" with
numerology. And yet, even within such a context, the reader who
takes seriously Boccaccio's poetics as revealed in the final books
of his *Genealogia* can sense in the pyrotechnics of the numbers "game"
a quasi-serious allusion to the spiritual blindness of the *brigata*. All
numerological signs appear to point to the presence of a triune God
and of the labors involved in the seven days of creation (or in observing the seven virtues). Yet the *brigata* will choose to prepare for
ten days of festivities intended to forget the almost apocalyptic
destruction that is ravaging the city. It is important to note that
the numerological frame comes into play immediately following
the description of the plague and before the decision to take flight. [13]

If we then consider that the group has gathered in Santa Maria
Novella — at this time the center of the university and of the hospital
facilities of Florence — and that among their more serious concerns
while in church is the fact that all they can really do is to count
cadavers as they arrive for burial, or to decide whether the friars
of the church were chanting their offices at the appropriate hours,
or indeed to display the quality and quantity of their sorrows by
means of their black attire, we begin to feel terribly jarring effects.
First, we note that the *brigata*'s actions and decisions are reminiscent of the inhuman behavior of the city people — a mode of conduct which extends to the narrator's obviously ironical defense of
their behavior by claiming that the exceptional laxity of all laws
fully justified the *brigata*'s decision to spend two pleasurable weeks
away from the infection. Secondly, their hedonistic argument that
they were free to do as they pleased provided they hurt no one was
specious to say the least, especially under the circumstances. And
thirdly, the obviously astounding behavior of the three young men
who, like dandies, are wandering around town to get a glimpse
of their girlfriends marks the group as a whole as one whose motives
are highly questionable whether in a Christian or simply human
context. While to a modern reader the *brigata*'s desire for pleasure
and enjoyment may appear practical and praiseworthy, for readers

who had experienced the plague firsthand their actions could only be viewed as contemptible.

There are a number of signs to indicate that all is not right with the *brigata*. There is first of all the narrator's decision to withhold the true names of its female constituency. "I could tell you their actual names, but refrain from doing so for a good reason, namely that I would not want any of them to feel embarrassed, at any time in the future, on account of the ensuing stories, all of which they either listened to or narrated themselves. For nowadays, laws relating to pleasure are somewhat restrictive."[14]

The behavior of the group as it organizes its fifteen-day sojourn contains certain features which likewise bear careful scrutiny. We learn at the outset of the uneasiness of certain of its members over some of the suggestions presented, then of the obvious luxuriousness of the surroundings to which they retire, and finally of the equivocal conditions set forth by Dioneo.

All are eager to adopt Pampinea's proposal to change the predicament of the seven young ladies from one of fear and apprehension to one which would allow "whatever pleasures and entertainments the present time will afford." Her argument includes the following principal points:

1. The preservation of one's life is a natural right and cannot be wrong since it harms no one;

2. All they have been able to do is to go to church and observe the misbehavior, illnesses, and deaths of their townsfolk;

3. Even at home they are faced with empty households bereft above all of servants;

4. Everyone with private means such as theirs has departed;

5. Most of their friends and relatives have died.

She therefore suggests that they go to one of their country estates where life can be much more pleasant without the frightening scenes of sickness and death. If they "do nothing" it will mean distress and mourning and the possible forfeit of their lives.

Following the first surge of enthusiasm, however, some doubts are raised by two of the ladies. Filomena expresses concern about the irrationality and disorganization of women without men. Elissa concurs but expresses doubts about the availability of men since most of their menfolk are dead. Total strangers are not feasible as companions because "wherever we go for our pleasure and repose, no trouble or scandal should come of it."

When the three men enter the scene it is Neifile who expresses concern about possible public censure if they invite the men along. But Filomena declares, "If I live honestly and my conscience is clear, then people may say whatever they like. . . . "[15] Whereupon all the necessary preparations for the journey to a hideaway are rapidly concluded, and the next day (a Wednesday, the mercurial point of the week) the men and women set forth with a retinue of servants for one of their estates, a mere two miles from Florence: "The spot in question was some distance away from any road, on a small hill that was agreeable to behold for its abundance of shrubs and trees, all bedecked in green leaves. . . . Delectable gardens and meadows lay all around, and there were wells of cool, refreshing water. The cellars were stocked with precious wines, more suited to the palates of connoisseurs than to sedate and respectable ladies."[16] As though to round off clearly the spirit that is to dominate the enforced sojourn, Dioneo, at the first general gathering, makes it known that the group must either totally forget Florence and the plague and agree to laugh and amuse itself or he will go back. Pampinea agrees forthwith and proposes that they organize themselves to assure the attainment of such a goal. For this suggestion she is crowned Queen of the first day by Filomena, and in instructing the servants she orders that nothing but cheerful news be allowed throughout the stay. The *brigata* then disperses until mealtime "talking of pleasant matters, weaving garlands of different leaves and singing love songs." Following an elaborate dinner the group dances and sings to the accompaniment of musical instruments, creating a scene clearly intended as contrast to the atrocious sufferings of the plague.

This detailed description of the manner in which the tales of the *Decameron* are introduced leaves little doubt that the central motif must be "escape from menace," to borrow a phrase used by Charles Singleton many years ago.[17] Why would Boccaccio choose to open his masterpiece in this fashion? To call it artistic strategy intended to provide a compelling rationale for his frame story is simply not sufficient since the question remains as to why the plague and not some other more pleasant pretext is selected for the *brigata*'s two-week sojourn in the country, especially since the behavior of the *brigata* is so reminiscent of the tradition of the "courts of love" with their emphasis on pleasant social intercourse. Why, then, the plague, if not to provide an ironical and contrapuntal beat to each moment of the evolving structure of the whole, a beat which sets the tone and perspective suggested by the double title, *The Ten Days or Prince Galehaut*? If the author is indeed trying to help "fair ladies in love" to avoid becoming victims of their lovesickness, then the revolting scenes of non-love presented in the description of the plague cry out against all forms of love — from the frailty of human devotion to the frailty of all human values and institutions that can be easily and quickly destroyed. In short, the plague in the *Decameron* resembles the voice of Augustine in Petrarch's *Secretum* reminding his protégé not only of the fragility of the human condition but of the fearfulness of the final moment of life and of the evanescent nature of human love. This sort of statement is hardly conducive to alleviating the lovesickness of young ladies.

Before proceeding further we must ask ourselves who is the narrator of the *Proem* and the *Introduction*. The obvious answer would appear to be Boccaccio himself. The possibility nevertheless remains that it could be the author's *persona*, for this same situation seems to hold in all his minor works: in these writings, scholars have sought in vain to identify Boccaccio personally behind the masks of a variety of narrators or protagonists.[18] All we *really* know is that in the opening of the *Decameron* we have a writer who is writing shortly after Florence was devastated by the plague in 1348, and that he is a writer who has somehow managed to become once again a free man by escaping from the clutches of a destructive love. He displays no gratitude whatsoever for having himself somehow escaped the plague. Failure to see a *persona* other than Boccaccio personally as the *moi* of the frame has led to a distortion of perspective in reading the great work. It might indeed be noted that as the *brigata* is introduced the narrator distances himself still more from the frame by remarking that the account of why, when and where the *brigata* met had been passed on to him by a "persona degna di fede." The narrator is therefore recounting not something he knew, but something he heard, and he can therefore afford to create an ironical distance between his own account of the plague and the behavior of the *brigata*. This is emphasized further in the *Conclusion* where the narrator insists that if some of the stories appear unattractive it is not his fault, for ". . . I could only transcribe the stories as they were actually told, which means that if the ladies who told them had told them better, I should have written them better." He then adds, "But even if one could assume that I was the inventor as well as the scribe of these stories (which was not the case) . . . ,"[19] he would still not feel ashamed that they were not beautiful, for only God is perfect. In this last citation we actually see Boccaccio himself distinguishing between "lo inventore e lo scrittore" as well as disclaiming the actual authorship.

From this perspective it is possible to maintain that the reason the narrator feels compelled to include the horrors of the plague in his opening is to contrast the experience through which he intends to put his lovesick ladies to that of the *brigata*. By comparing the appalling scenes of the plague to a climb of a steep and rugged mountain and assuring his ladies that only in this way can they truly find the ensuing plain easy and pleasurable to traverse, the narrator is preparing us for the strange behavior of the *brigata* which implies that its members had failed to undertake such a climb and thus are not to be envied or admired but rather to be viewed with scepticism and suspicion. Starting with the artificial self-organization of the *brigata* and proceeding to the sequence of days, of stories, of festivities and of commentaries the alert reader must be constantly wary of each member of the *brigata*. It would be easy to admire and even sympathize with their actions, but this is precisely why the book may be another Prince Galehaut. The many signs, numerological and otherwise, that surrounded the formation of the *brigata* must not go unheeded. Nor must the manner in which the group caters to Dioneo, the wise libertine, and to his bawdy tales.

Dioneo's insistence on reserving the tenth story of the last nine days for himself makes such tales particularly significant inasmuch as they represent the only perfectly free moments of storytelling. Dioneo's stories are not restricted by any rules or conventions and are thus more indicative of the true nature of the *brigata* than are those of the other narrators who must abide by the theme set for each day. The group's penchant for laughing at Fortune or at man's inhumanity can easily be admired as the healthy perspective of wise people, but a close look reveals that it is the laughter of fools. The significantly-spaced stories of Ciappelletto (No. 1), Fra Rustico (No. 30), and Don Gianni (No. 90) are perhaps the best examples of how absolute evil is quite capable of producing laughter.

In summary, as we move from the *Proem* to the opening of Day
I we are made to recall the masterpieces of Dante and Petrarch
in their deepest significance as well as the writings of St. Augustine
and Boethius. The *brigata* is the exemplification of the false good
whose self-centeredness is the exact opposite of Christian doctrine
and life. We do indeed have the depiction of an extremely broad
segment of humanity throughout the tales, but the reaction to
humanity's behavior and actions must be viewed from the perspective of the devastating plague which, as a super-symbol of death
itself, can never be escaped but must instead be met head-on with
the full knowledge that the final accounting will be calculated by
an infallible mind and not by those who, like the *brigata*, are will-
ing to take their chances. The reaction of the *brigata* to each story
as well as their general comportment are not to be accepted or im-
itated offhandedly, but rather to be meditated upon and digested,
for the group's behavior reveals a great deal about the extent to
which its members are indulging in what Berchorius, a contemporary of Boccaccio, considers one of the greatest spiritual dangers
of springtime — "the chattering of words and foolish mirth."[20]

For the alert reader the simultaneous closeness and distance of
the plague provides a kind of death rattle in the laughter of the
brigata and of the casual readers who see humor in the scenes of
man's inhumanity to man. Such readers are indeed running the
risk of being victimized by their blind enjoyment of the book, and
in choosing to disregard the danger signaled by the subtitle of the
work they remind all readers that the work might be a pander for
the devil and might lead to a death and damnation reminiscent
of the plague. In short, we must learn to read the *Decameron* with
the realization that ultimately it encompasses both a theory of life
and theory of literature as envisioned by St. Augustine and as
developed by Boethius, Dante and Petrarch in their masterpieces
and by Boccaccio in the last two books of his *Genealogia*. In order
to grasp this rich heritage one must start paying closer attention
to such signposts as the subtitle, the *Proem*, the plague, the behavior
of the *brigata* and the role of the narrator.

Having seen the signs to the alert reader scattered throughout
the *Proem* and *Introduction*, let us turn next to the *Introduction to the
Fourth Day*. Its main thrust is really directed against the accusation
that Boccaccio is excessively involved with his "vaghe donne." All
too often the parable of the hermit father and son recited by Boccaccio at this point in his defense is interpreted as a defense of

naturalism. There are, however, simply too many observations added by Boccaccio to the parable to leave it at that. One might even
note that the ladies who attract the boy's attention are far from being provocative or sensuously appealing in their personal appearance. Instead they are in a *brigata* which is returning from a
wedding, and are elegantly attired. The boy's desire to bring one
home is therefore prompted by their beauty which as he notes is
superior to the painted angels that his father had often shown him.
He indeed finds it inconceivable that such beauty could contain
evil, as his father implies. Its similarity to the powers of feminine
beauty in v,1 where a near-savage is converted into a highly
cultivated person through his contact with and desire for such beauty
begs for acknowledgment. As for the play on the feeding of the "gos-
lings," it is in the minds of the father and of the reader that the
sexual overtones are to be recognized, and not in the mind of the
boy. It is significant that the half-tale is immediately followed by
the observation of the author concerning the two functions of
women. On the one hand they provide physical and sexual
pleasures, but on the other they afford the delight of having seen
and of seeing continuously ". . . graceful elegance, . . . endearing
charm, and . . . enchanting beauty, to say nothing of . . . womanly
decorum." If such creatures could be so pleasing to "a witless youth,"
how could critics blame the author for striving to please them?

The subsequent references to Guido Cavalcanti, Dante and Cino
da Pistoia, as well as to many others throughout history, as examples of great men who had even in old age continued to strive
eagerly to please ladies, likewise seem to stress the inspirational
and aesthetic qualities of lovely women rather than their powers
of merely satisfying the appetites. Indeed the implication that such
ladies are at but a single remove from the Muses themselves, and
are not therefore distractions from the inspirations of Parnassus
further defines the positive value of his "vaghe donne" who, like
the young hermit boy, have yet to learn the potentially explosive
nature of human love and indeed of the human condition. In the
"fables" written specifically for them such youths will find "more
bread than many a rich man in his treasures." To love and serve
truly beautiful women does not thwart the laws of nature, and if
his detractors prefer to live in their kinds of pleasure (which are
referred to as "appetiti corrotti"), let them at least allow him to live
in his kind which by extension are neither "appetiti" nor "corrotti."
The subsequent tales of Day IV with their tragic loves and the con-

stant pall of death remind us rather of the plague than of the enjoyment men can have with "papere." The tales of Day IV clearly show the deadly seriousness of Boccaccio's defense of his art which opens Day IV.

Boccaccio's final justification of the *Decameron* occurs in the *Conclusion*. Addressing once again his "vaghe donne" he expresses first the hope that he had indeed afforded them the consolation promised and then announces his intention to supplement his defense of the fourth day with further remarks directed against possible and anticipated criticisms.

The first criticism deals with the possibility that he had used excessive license ". . . in that I have sometimes caused ladies to say, and very often to hear, things which are not very suitable to be heard or said by virtuous women."[21] His response is that even the most unchaste matters can be handled chastely by the use of proper language. Furthermore, even were the charge true, the contents of the stories required it. Only those who view them with a "ragionevole occhio" could appreciate the inextricability of form and content. What is more, the stories are being told not in church nor in school, but in gardens and in a "luogo di sollazzo" among fully mature people who could not be led astray by stories, and at a time when "even the most respectable people saw nothing unseemly in wearing their breeches over their heads if they thought their lives might be preserved"[22] — a glancing barb against human selfishness in the face of the plague.

In short, the contents could be either harmful or useful depending upon the listener or reader just as with wine, fire or arms whose effects depend on their use. No corrupt mind ever understands words healthily, nor can a well-disposed mind be harmed by words that are somewhat less than proper. Even sacred Scripture had sent people to perdition by being perversely understood. A writer must consider his audience. Idle ladies in love could hardly be expected to enjoy reading matter of high seriousness in a lofty and pithy style. As for the excessive jests and jokes, they too are intended for particular effects — especially the retention of the interest of ladies whose melancholy must be driven away. Thus does Boccaccio reach the "desiderato fine" of his work. He feels that he has indeed afforded solace to women in love!

What then is the meaning of Boccaccio's four intrusions as found in the *Proem*, the *Introduction to Day I*, the *Introduction to Day IV* and the *Conclusion*? Is it mere rhetoric? Why would his "idle ladies" re-

quire such interruptions? Could it be that perhaps we should recon-
sider who or what the "gentilissime donne" may be? Could Boccaccio really be offering such young ladies a sop to their lovesickness?
I would suggest that the term "beautiful women" refers to pure souls
in battle with the flesh who are mature enough to feel the frailty
of the human condition with its incredible complexity, and who
need the periodic voice of reason to remind them that the road to
salvation is truly difficult and fraught with danger.[23] The reaction
of the *brigata* to its own tales is not to be trusted by the alert reader
for they do indeed seem to be telling them as mere pastimes, as
a means of postponing the necessary climb.[24] In fact they feel free
to tell even the most bawdy tales presumably because of the total
lack of moral restraints caused by the plague. It was precisely for
this reason that the author had felt obliged to assign fictitious names
to them. Their carefully-organized miniature society, with its air
of aristocratic sophistication, is interested only in a reality created
exclusively for its personal gratification. But since the roots of such
a reality were firmly anchored in the horrors of the plague, the
group's hedonism had to reflect a moral and spiritual truancy that
was readily recognizable by any reader aware of the Christian ethic.
It is this second level of reality that the "vaghe donne" to whom
the work is dedicated are expected to grasp and to learn from. It
is the reality that exists only for those who can view the plague
as God's signal of what earthly life ultimately means. In a sense
it is the world of unchanging values whose existence many of the
tales actually reinforce by denying it, as in the very first tale. Like
Dante's musician friend, Casella, in *Purgatorio* II, the *brigata* tells
tales "come a nessun toccasse altro la mente," but the voice of God
in the form of the plague and of the author's four intrusions is, like
Dante's Cato, a constant reminder of what could befall unwary
readers accustomed to read as did Paolo and Francesca, so clearly
recalled in the subtitle. In many ways, Boccaccio's intrusions could
be viewed as counterpoints to the plague.

What does such an awareness by the alert reader do to the reading
of the stories themselves? Does it afford greater unity to such
reading, or does it spoil it for those who simply want to enjoy the
stories on their most superficial level with their simplistic view of
man in all his potential? Let us see.

It is unlikely that the first three stories could be of any interest
to fair ladies in love. Ciappelletto's sleazy activities, Abraham's conversion, and wealthy Melchizedek's wise answer to the Saladin

could hardly be expected to entertain such ladies as might the fourth tale which speaks of lust among friars. The same may be said of the sermon-like tales 6 through 8 of the first day as compared with tales 9 and 10 with their flattery of female power. What, therefore, is there about the first day that might have had the desired impact on the "vaghe donne?" All tales but the first are surprisingly brief, and all ten seem to address a complex human situation requiring the use of wit, knowledge or wisdom in order to disentangle it. Each of the tales also deals with persons of high state, except No. 1. What indeed can we make of No. 1 which occupies such a strategic position according to medieval canons of art? In my opinion the first tale stands with respect to the entire *Decameron* as Canto I stands in relation to the whole *Divine Comedy*.

Accepting Branca's three broad themes which underpin the *Decameron*, namely, Fortune, Love and Wit, the first and last are certainly writ large in the tale of Ciappelletto. A disastrous undertaking on which Fortune seems to have turned her back is salvaged in the very face of death through the diabolical use of wit. Even the theme of love assumes universal though negative proportions in Ciappelletto's sacrilegious display of charity. If the conclusion of the tale reflects an overflow of divine charity, Ciappelletto is a perfect exemplar of the Antichrist. When misused, Fortune, Wit and Love are but perversions of Faith, Hope and Charity. What we therefore have in the first tale is a summary statement of the whole work with a satanic figure, as in Dante, being as thoroughly duped as he thought he had duped his fellow men and his Creator. As Branca's three themes begin to unfold in Day I we slowly begin to witness how the forces they represent could be used or abused. Whether Saladin, abbot, inquisitor, king or other ruler, or just common man, all are subject to the blindness that so often makes human beings fall prey to one or more of these forces.

A moment's reflection would show that Ciappelletto's "heroic" confession and demise are but the equivalent of the self-centered actions of the Florentines in the face of death during the plague, including the behavior of the *brigata* which, like Ciappelletto in the face of misfortune, tries so foolishly to create perfection out of chaos and misfortune through the use of wit and ingenuity. On the surface, of course, it appears as though Ciappelletto is really the victor; but this would mean that he had succeeded in making a fool of God. If read carefully, the ending of the story actually reveals just the opposite meaning. According to Panfilo, the narrator, it is most likely that Ciappelletto's soul must be in hell. If so, then God's love must be infinite since He had allowed such a monstrous sinner to act as his intermediary simply because the sinner had convinced everyone through his confessors that he was a saint. We thus have a truly diabolical act of fraud against the Creator being miraculously converted into an act of divine charity. Panfilo's clear gloss could not be simpler.[25]

We may conclude therefore that, like Dante in the presence of Satan, we too must shift our perspective in order to grasp Boccaccio's strangely moral universe. The outwitting of Fortune or of one's rival in the battle of love can elicit our compassion or even our admiration. The attempt to outwit one's Creator, however, is foolhardy indeed, and we must be careful before we laugh too heartily, for we may be abusing what we should really be using for our edification, namely, human wit whose proper perspective must never confuse which end is up and which down.

This perspective clearly prevails in the tales of Day II devoted to adventures having unexpectedly happy endings. Only through such a perspective can a reader perceive that all of the endings are highly materialistic, consisting either of acquiring unexpected riches (as in eight of the tales) or of being undeservedly saved from a dangerous situation (as in the first and the last tales). The entire day seems to be dedicated to extolling Lady Fortune — an activity fraught with danger to the medieval mind.

The alert reader will also note that in the third day what the protagonists gain or regain is lustful pleasure. Day IV with its introductory parable of the young boy, as was already noted, shows the fatality of love as a passion: seven tales ending with the death of both lovers, two with lovers barely escaping death, and one with a desperate beloved becoming a nun.

By the end of Day IV any innocent lady in love or pure soul trying to remain pure must feel a sense of bewilderment at the depictions of the human race in battle with the mysterious powers of Fortune or Amor. Suddenly one senses relief in the resolutions of the tales of Day V. The griefs and misfortunes of basic human passions and the interactions of men in society are overcome by the simple measure of having recourse to a holy sacrament — matrimony.[26] In this sacrament may be discerned the manner in which man can resolve his battle with those mysterious forces of Fortune, Wit and Love that seem to have such a grip on him as a member of society. From the power of beauty and love in the first story we move through the powers of constancy, chastity, prudence, religion and devotion, and finally to Dioneo's last tale of a depraved marriage. The nature of the tales, the careful balancing of the parts, and even the very language has understandably prompted Mario Fubini to call Day V "la giornata della poesia." The world of intrigue and deceit with its echoes of the horrors of the plague seems suddenly to end with Day V. But here too, at the beginning of Dioneo's tenth tale, we find an image that, like the tale of Ciappelletto, turns out to be terribly misleading to the unwary reader. His advice to the listening *brigata* is this: "While you listen to it, do as you do when you enter a garden and, stretching out your delicate hands, pluck the roses and avoid the thorns." He then concludes: "In doing so, leave the bad man in his misfortune with his woes, and laugh at the amorous tricks of his wife,"[27] advice which reminds us that Dionysian forces will ever be present to undermine even the most respected institutions. Both husband and wife are clearly depraved.

As we turn to Day VI we encounter that other dimension of life — not man as he is subject to external forces but man, isolated, as he is subject to internal ones. Here too man's awesome ability to use his powers of language and intellect to victimize his fellow men reminds us of Ciappelletto's dark victory as well as the grim behavior of the Florentines during the plague. To recognize the proper and improper uses of such personal powers is vital.

Day VI with its witty *motti* and extreme brevity seems to reflect a certain innocent use of such powers. The alert reader must nevertheless take careful note of the casual half-tale that introduces Day VI in which we witness a brief altercation between two of the servants regarding the virginity of women in and out of wedlock. Dioneo's resolution of the argument once again suggests the unlikelihood that fallen man can regain much of his lost innocence.

On the other hand, in Day VII, which has been called the triumph of adultery, we witness a series of womanly wiles used to cuckold husbands. Despite its beauty and symmetry the Valley of the Ladies to which the *brigata* moves for Day VII becomes indeed a kind of unkempt den of lust as the stories unfold. Just as the Valley is located at the furthest point from the plague with its suffering humanity, so do the stories achieve a new low in moral degeneracy since they depict the denigration of a sacrament. Likewise Day VIII is full of tales of venal love and uncharitable behavior as men and women try to outwit one another. Day VII and Day VIII clearly echo Day

III and Day II respectively with each set of stories proclaiming either the inhumanity or the bestiality of man. Day IX echoes Day I in being a free day with no specific subject matter for the tales. In sharp contrast to Day I, however, Day IX contains tales that really show the frightening and callous way in which people can deal with one another, under the guise of good faith. While the general spirit may be comic, it is reminiscent of the dark humor encountered in the tale of Ciappelletto. It is epitomized in the tenth tale of Dioneo who tells of the "brilliant" trick played by a priest in helping a gullible husband convert his wife into a mare by pinning a "tail" on her. The opening and close of this last tale of Day IX (as in the first tale of Day I) contain some rather clear signals concerning the way to read Boccaccio's masterpiece. In introducing his tale Dioneo proclaims: "Charming ladies, the beauty of a flock of white doves is better enhanced by a black crow than by a pure white swan; and likewise the presence of a simpleton among a group of intelligent people will sometimes add brilliance and grace to their wisdom, as well as affording pleasure and amusement. Accordingly, since you are all models of tact and discretion, whereas I am something of a fool, I ought to command a higher place in your affections, by augmenting the light of your excellence through my own shortcomings, than if I were to diminish it by my superior worth. And hence, in telling you the story I am about to relate, I must claim greater licence to present myself in my true colours, and crave your more patient indulgence, than if I were blessed with greater intelligence."[28]

These rather strange observations seem to echo Dioneo's words at the end of Day VI just before assuming the crown as ruler of the following day. There in response to the ladies' objections that his suggested topic for Day VII is ill-befitting them, Dioneo responds: "What you point out is powerless to make me change my command, in view of the fact that the times are such that any kind of talk is allowed, provided men and women abstain from wrongdoing. You know that owing to the misery of the times the judges have deserted the tribunals, the laws both human and divine are silent, and full license is granted everyone to save his own life. So, if you enlarge your chastity (Onestà) a little in talk, not to follow it with immodest actions but to amuse yourselves and others, I do not see how anyone in the future can find any plausible reason for condemning you."[29] Such is the chastity of the ladies that if it did not fail at the threat of death, it certainly would not do so by listening to a few merry tales. Indeed if anyone learned that they had refrained from talking about such trifles he might assume that the ladies were suffering from guilty consciences. Therefore, Dioneo concludes, "Put off a suspicion more befitting evil minds than yours, and let everyone think of a good tale to tell." The subsequent move to the breathtaking Valley of the Ladies offers an environment in striking contrast to the bawdy actions of the adulterous heroines of the stories. The atmosphere is strongly reminiscent of the distinction Berchorius made between spring as a time of penance and a time of danger when "all animals are stimulated to desire, in which birds delight to chatter, to fly and to play," a time signifying "worldly prosperity . . . in which abound the urge of desire and lust, chattering of words and foolish mirth." The Valley is a perfect garden of love where the ladies' chastity is indeed "enlarged."[30]

The move to the Valley represents the furthest point reached by the *brigata* in its desire to avoid human intercourse with the outside world. Similarly Dioneo's tenth tale of Day IX seems to reflect the lowest point to which men's actions could sink. Not only does the priest-protagonist, Don Gianni, deceive close friends, but in doing so knowingly feigns practicing magic against the very sacrament that, as we saw, is intended to be the most divine binding force in society — matrimony. We thus see a man of God (not a friar) not only ridiculing the bonds of marriage, but in the eyes of the simple couple possessing the power to convert a wife into an animal. If Ciappelletto's was an unforgivable crime against God, Don Gianni's is an unforgivable crime against both God and man. The reaction of Dioneo's female audience to the tale makes one wonder not only about the extent to which they have indeed "enlarged" their chastity, but whether there is any remnant of charity left in them: "They laughed as if they were never going to stop at this tale, which was better understood by the ladies than Dioneo had intended." It is at this point that the wary reader begins to grasp why the "vaghe donne" forming the *real* audience might indeed "better understand" than the ladies of the *brigata* who seemed so forgetful of the plague and so open to the "chattering of words and foolish mirth" encouraged by Dioneo.

Day X seems naturally to provide badly needed relief for the mysterious tensions of the second half of the *Decameron* just as Day V had done for the first half. In the topic and stories of Day X the message emerges that, just as in the first half, matrimony provides a peaceful spiritual resolution for man's endless struggle with the chaotic forces that seem to impel him externally, in like manner does virtuous behavior provide the needed antidote for the explosive forces residing inside him. And, as the ruler of the last day, Panfilo remarks that it is man's awareness of his own mortality that prompts him to aspire to lofty actions. The first three stories reflect the workings of internal forces among opposing types of individuals at the very highest levels of society, whether in the West among kingly nobility (tale 1), or among the highest church circles (tale 2), or in the Far East among its legendary wise men (tale 3). Whether a victim of pride (tale 1), anger (tale 2) or envy (tale 3), man possesses the capacity for overcoming these negative impulses by practicing Charity.

In tales 4–7 we see a virtuous act resolve the strife caused by self-centeredness in affairs of the heart. In tales 8–9 we observe how virtue begets virtue in unbelievably complicated interactions of internal forces. Finally in tale 10 we observe how the supreme virtue of an understanding heart serves as a bond in marriage despite the prevalence of Fortune and Wit as despotic powers.

Matrimony and Virtue as the two great stabilizing forces in society and in the individual thus seem to divide in two Boccaccio's great masterpiece. This pattern emerges, however, only through careful reading and despite the truant "mirth" of the *brigata* whose most significant member (Fiammetta) in the very final song continues to bemoan her misfortunes in love and her mistrust of all men and women. The confused and chaotic spirit of the opening thus seems to be restored as the *brigata* prepares to leave. Indeed even before Fiammetta's song Panfilo gives as the three soundest reasons for returning to Florence (1) the possibility that the companions' stay in the country may become boring, (2) the risk of petty arguments and (3) the possibility that others may try to break into their closed circle. In reviewing the *brigata*'s experience Panfilo notes: "As you know, it will be a fortnight tomorrow since we left Florence to find some amusement to support our health and vitality and to escape the melancholy, agony and woes which have continued in our city since the beginning of the plague."[31] In his opinion the *brigata* had acted most virtuously, for despite the merry tales which perhaps might incline to concupiscence, despite the eating and drinking, the playing and the singing, "all of which things incite weak minds to things less than serious," he had noticed nothing but continual virtue, concord and fraternal familiarity among its members. When on the following day the *brigata* returns to Florence no mention whatsoever is made of the plague or its ravages. This silence dramatizes the extent to which the *brigata* was unconcerned about the horrors of the plague, except on the level of self-preservation. Having returned to Santa Maria Novella, "the three young men went off in search of other diversions; and in due course the ladies returned to their homes."[32]

Even for the most unsophisticated reader the *brigata* could never be viewed as having acted in an exemplary fashion with respect to the plague. Its very members considered its greatest accomplishment the extent to which they had succeeded in enjoying themselves despite the plague. Notwithstanding its presumably virtuous conduct during the fortnight of merriment, its self-centeredness and desire to avoid contact with other humans — even unafflicted ones — could hardly be called charitable. Nor could its choice of questionable subject matter which might incline to concupiscence and which called for the "enlargement of chastity" be viewed as anything but folly. Pampinea's effective organization of the activities of the participants allowed absolutely no time for truly individual meditation. Even during the so-called holy days no reference whatsoever is made to prayers or services for the dying thousands. There is little doubt, therefore, that for a reader to view the tales as "useful and virtuous" or as offering "utility and good fruits" he or she could not overlook the role and behavior of the *brigata*, especially if he or she had lived through the horror of the plague.

Boccaccio must certainly have been acquainted with Petrarch's letter to his brother Gerardo (*Fam.* XVI, 2), a Carthusian monk, in which Petrarch expresses the pride he felt at his brother's comportment during the height of the same plague. According to the account reaching Petrarch in Padua, Gerardo, determined to remain firm in the place assigned to him by Christ, had refused to obey his Prior's order to abandon the monastery and had remained behind with thirty-four ill members of the community. The Prior died a few days after returning home, but Gerardo saw all of the thirty-four die despite his assistance, and gave each a proper burial. He subsequently succeeded in reconstituting the religious community, prompting Petrarch to observe, "And so you returned as if to found a second time your venerable monastery made barren by death and guarded and defended by your faith and your wise chastity."

If we now return to the *Decameron* and try to determine what distinguishes the behavior of Boccaccio's *brigata* from the general run of the phantom-like figures that remained to face the horrors of the plague the answer must be the ingenuity of the young people not only in avoiding contact with the pestilence but in enjoying themselves thoroughly during those terrible days. That Boccaccio could possibly have been extolling such behavior is hardly likely in view of the spirit of Petrarch's letter which represented the position of the true intellectual in the face of such calamities.

If therefore the stories are to be read for "utility and good fruits," and if the book is not going to serve as a pander for evil, the alert reader must be sensitive to many things, but especially to the key lessons provided by the frame of the work. There is first the lesson that emerges from the chief purpose of the book as stated by the author in the *Proem*; second, the lesson reflected in the behavior of the *brigata* in the face of the plague; third, the lesson inherent in the angry outcries of the author in defense of his art, and finally, the lesson emerging from the obvious symmetrical patterns that neatly divide the work into two parts. But the primary sensitivity of the alert reader must be to the plague which serves throughout the book as a silent reminder of the precariousness of the human condition. As Dante's *Comedy* had taught, the dividing line between damnation and salvation may be very fine indeed.

notes

1. Robert Hollander, *Boccaccio's Two Venuses* (New York, 1977), p. 6. The search for unity has, however, been sporadic and inconclusive as a result of dealing separately with each section of the total frame. In many ways the extremes of interpretation were most clearly defined for English scholars when, in 1944, Charles Singleton took sharp exception with Angelo Lipari's attempt to find a *sovrasenso* which he felt was the real meaning of the work. The two positions were expressed in Charles S. Singleton, "On Meaning in the Decameron," *Italica* 21 (1944): 117–24 and Angelo Lipari, "Meaning and Real Significance of the *Decameron*," in H. M. Peyre, ed., *Essays in Honor of Albert Feuillerat, Yale Romanic Studies* 22 (1943): 43–83. The possibility of a *sovrasenso*, which Singleton found repugnant, found no supporters, but the principle of unity which informs the work continues to have many adherents who have generally insisted on the naturalistic quality of that unity, viewing it as a realistic depiction of the human condition in its infinite aspects. Other scholars, while accepting the naturalistic view, have also seen a moral force involved in the unifying principle.

Among the former may be cited Giovanni Getto, *Vita di forme e forme di vita nel 'Decameron'* (Milano, 1966); Aldo Scaglione, *Nature and Love in the Middle Ages* (Berkeley, 1963); Bruno Maier in his introduction to the works of Boccaccio (Bologna, 1967); Rafaello Ramat, "Indicazioni per una lettura del 'Decameron'," in *Saggi sul Rinascimento* (Firenze, 1969); Mario Baratti, *Realtà e stile nel 'Decameron'* (Vicenza, 1970); Giorgio Padoan, "Mondo aristocratico e mondo comunale nell'ideologia e nell'arte di Giovanni Boccaccio," *Studi sul Boccaccio* 2 (1964): 81–216.

Leading those critics who see the structure of the *Decameron* reflecting a moral concern is Vittore Branca whose *Boccaccio medioevale* (Firenze, 1956, 1970) set the stage for the global approach to Boccaccio's masterpiece. Others include Giuseppe Mazzotta, "The *'Decameron'*: The Marginality of Literature," *University of Toronto Quarterly* 42 (1972): 66–81, and "The *Decameron*: The Literal and the Allegorical," *Italian Quarterly* 18 (1975): 53–73; Mario Marti, "Interpretazione del *Decameron*," in *Dal certo al vero* (Rome, 1962); Giorgio Barberi Squarotti, "La 'cornice' del *Decameron* o il mito di Robinson," in *Da Dante al Novecento* (Milano, 1970); Joan M. Ferrante, "The Frame Characters of the *Decameron*: A Progression of Virtues," *Romance Philology* 19 (1965): 212–26; Robert Hollander, *Boccaccio's Two Venuses*, Chap. 4; Janet Levarie Smarr, "Symmetry and Balance in the *Decameron*," *Medaevalia* 2 (1976): 159–87. A middle position was most recently expressed by Lucia Marino in *The Decameron 'Cornice,'* (Ravenna, 1979).

2. "Comincia il libro chiamato Decameron, cognominato precipe Galeotto, nel quale si contengono cento novelle in diece dì dette da sette donne e da tre giovani uomini." All Italian citations are from V. Branca, *Decameron* (Milano, 1976) while the English translations are taken either from that of G. H. McWilliam, Penguin Classics (Middlesex, 1976) or from that of Richard Aldington (New York, 1949).

3. See Hollander, *Boccaccio's Two Venuses*, p. 102 for a discussion of the embarrassment the subtitle has caused critics. His observations on p. 101 on the manner in which the "Galeotto motif" had become a trope in Boccaccio's minor works support my position, as does his subsequent discussion on pp. 103–6. See also the incredible statement of Giorgio Padoan in his *Il Baccaccio, le Muse, il Parnaso, e l'Arno* (Firenze, 1978), p. 31 in which to distinguish the difference between Dante's position and Boccaccio's, he states: "Nell'intitolazione boccacciana invece svanisce ogni sottinteso polemico ed anzi, se mai, appare nello scrittore un certo compiacimento nell'essere 'Galeotto'. . . ."

4. "Umana cosa è avere compassione degli afflitti. . . ." Branca considers these opening words part of a rhetorical formula having widespread use in the Middle Ages. V. Branca, *Decameron*, p. 976. See, however, Dante's commentary on the sonnet of *Vita nuova* XV, ". . . in the last I say why people should have compassion . . ." on his sufferings for love.

5. V. Branca, *Decameron*, p. 977, n. 2; with greater detail in *Boccaccio medioevale*, pp. 300–32, which appears in English translation in the *Francesco*

Petrarca, Citizen of the World (Padua-Albany, 1980).

6. *Inf.* I, 8–9, trans. H. R. Huse (New York, 1954). "Ma per trattar del ben ch'io vi trovai / Dirò de l'altre cose ch'io vi ho scorte."

7. ". . . la mortifera pestilenza . . . per operazion de' corpi superiori o per le nostre inique opere da giusta ira di Dio a nostra correzione mandata sopra i mortali, alquanti anni davanti nelle parti orientali incominciata, quelle d'inumerabile quantità de' viventi avendo private, senza ristare d'un luogo in un altro continuandosi, verso l'Occidente miserabilmente s'era ampliata."

8. "E lasciamo stare che l'uno cittadino l'altro schifasse e quasi niuno vicino avesse dell'altro caro e i parenti insieme rade volte non mai si visitassero e di lontano."

9. ". . . l'un fratello l'altro abbandonava e il zio il nipote e la sorella il fratello e spesse volte la donna il suo marito, e, che maggior cosa è e quasi non credibile, li padri e le madri i figliuoli, quasi loro non fosser, di visitare e di servire schifavano."

10. ". . . infra 'l marzo e il prossimo luglio vegnente . . . oltre a centomila creature umane si crede per certo dentro alle mura della città di Firenze essere stati di vita tolti, che forse, anzi l'accidente mortifero, non si saria estimato tanti avervene dentro avuti."

11. In a recent article Gene Brucker presented historical evidence to prove that the Florentines faced the horrors and tensions of the Black Death with faith and courage rather than with hysteria or rash behavior. If the rather sparse evidence he presents is sufficient for generalization, it would appear that Boccaccio's description of the behavior of the Florentine populace is highly imaginative. If this is indeed the case, my thesis is considerabley strengthened. See Gene A. Brucker, "Florence and the Black Death," in Marga Cottino-Jones and Edward F. Tuttle, eds., *Boccaccio: Secoli di vita* (Ravenna, 1977), pp. 21–30. G. Padoan however seems to assume a kind of heroic stance by Boccaccio in the face of the plague: "Manca perciò accenno al tema più tipico e predominante del Medioevo, il *memento mori*. La moria è sconfitta non mediante il pentimento dei peccati e la pia preparazione all'al di là, ma con la riscossa delle ragioni della vita e della socialità," *Il Boccaccio, le Muse*, p. 47.

12. I am indebted to Bernard F. Huppé for these numerological indications. The role of numerology in Boccaccio's works is slowly being uncovered, particularly by the work of Victoria Kirkham who in a series of papers presented at various professional meetings has shown its extensiveness in several works of Boccaccio. See her "Reckoning with Boccaccio's 'questioni d'amore'," *Modern Language Notes* 89 (1974): 47–59. Also G. Padoan, *Il Boccaccio, le Muse*, chap. 1, for the evolution of Boccaccio's work following his move from Naples to Florence.

13. The following interpretation by Lucia Marino summarizes the usual attitude of critics toward this moment: "Significantly the *brigata*'s experience begins and ends in a church, a place of refuge from the world, of meditation and introspection. The *novellieri*'s inner transformation and renewal

occur through art and through peregrinations that are to be understood psychologically rather than in terms of spatial distance and topography. This profound insight of Boccaccio into the nature of art and the psychological healing and maturation processes explains . . . why an ideal bucolic cosmos suddenly appears in the midst of the earthly, plague-ravaged Tuscan *contado* . . . ," *The Decameron 'Cornice,'* p. 75. As will be shown, a careful reading of the author's words used to describe the *brigata*'s return to the city shows a total lack of charity or concern.

14. "Li nomi delle quali io in propria forma racconterei, se giusta cagione da dirlo non mi togliesse, la quale è questa: che io non voglio per le rac-contate cose da loro, che seguono, e per l'ascoltate nel tempo avvenire alcuna di loro possa prendere vergogna, essendo oggi alquanto ristrette le leggi al piacere. . . ."

15. ". . . là dove io onestamente viva nè mi rimorda d'alcuna cosa la coscienze, parli chi vuole in contrario."

16. ". . . sopra una piccola montagnetta, da ogni parte lontano alquanto alle nostre strade, di varii albuscelli e piante tutte di verdi fronde ripiene . . . con pratelli da torno e con giardini maravigliosi e con pozzi d'acque freschissime e con volte di preziosi vini: cose più atte a curiosi bevitori che a sobrie e oneste donne."

17. Singleton, "On Meaning in the *Decameron*," passim.

18. In *Boccaccio's Two Venuses*, pp. 107–8, Hollander offers what he calls a "brief morphology of the narrators" in ten of Boccaccio's works. He con-cludes that the narrators move from lovers in seven of the works, to a disenchanted lover in the *Elegia di Madonna Fiammetta*, to a freed lover in the *Decameron*, and to a misogynist in the *Corbaccio*. Thus in the last three works the narrator's expressed intent is to turn us away from love, while in the first seven it is "to celebrate the Amore to whom he himself is subject."

19. ". . . io non potè nè doveva scrivere se non le raccontate, e per ciò esse che le dissero le dovevan dir belle e io l'avrei scritte belle. . . . Ma se pur prosuppor si volesse che io fossi stato di quelle e lo inventore e lo scrittore, *che non fui* . . ."

20. Berchorius, *Reductorium morale*, "De quadragesima," V, xlvii, cited in Bernard F. Huppé, *A Reading of the Canterbury Tales* (Albany, 1964), pp. 19–20.

21. ". . . in fare alcuna volta dire alle donne e molto spesso ascoltare cose non assai convenienti nè a dire nè a ascoltare a oneste donne."

22. ". . . andar con le brache in capo per iscampo di sè era alli più onesti non disdicevole. . . ."

23. Janet Smarr, "Symmetry and Balance," p. 185, n. 29, suggests something similar.

24. See, however, Joan M. Ferrante, "The Frame Characters," p. 213, where each of the female narrators is identified with one of the seven vir-tues, and each of the males with "qualities which are also necessary to the proper development of the soul."

25. For an extreme, though intriguing, interpretation, see Millicent

Marcus, "Ser Ciappelletto: A Reader's Guide to the *Decameron*," *Humanities Association of Canada Bulletin* 26 (1977): 275–88.

26. For a slightly different analysis of the total structure, and particularly the centrality of Day V, see Janet Smarr, "Symmetry and Balance," passim.

27. "E voi, ascoltandola, quello ne fate che usate siete di fare quando ne' giardini entrate, che, distesa la dilicata mano, cogliete le rose e lasciate le spine stare. . . il che farete lasciando il cattivo uomo con la mala ventura stare con la sua disonestà, e liete riderete degli amorosi inganni della sua donna. . . ."

28. "Leggiadre donne, infra molte bianche colombe agiunge più di bellezza un nero corvo che non farebbe un candido cigno; e così tra molti savi alcuna volta un men savio è non solamente accrescere splendore e bellezza alla loro maturità, ma ancora diletto e sollazzo. Per la qual cosa, essendo voi tutte discretissime e moderate, io, il quale sento anzi dello scemo che no, faccendo la vostra virtù più lucente col mio difetto più vi debbo esser caro che se con più valore quella facessi divenire più oscura; e per conseguente più largo arbitrio debbo avere in dimostrarvi tal qual io sono, e più pazientemente debbo da voi esser sostenuto, che non dovrebbe se io più savio fossi. . . ."

29. ". . . da imporlo non mi potè istorre quello che voi me volete mostrare, pensando che il tempo è tale che, guardandosi e gli uomini e le donne l'operar disonestamente, ogni ragionare è conceduto. Or non sapete voi che, per la perversità di questa stagione, li giudici hanno lasciati i tribunali? le leggi, così le divine come le umane, tacciono? e ampia licenzia per conservar la vita è conceduta a ciascuno? Per che, se alquanto s'allarga la vostra onestà nel favellare, non per dover con l'opere mai alcuna cosa sconcia seguire ma per dar diletto a voi e a altrui, non veggio con che argomento da concedere vi possa nello avvenire riprendere alcuno."

30. For the Berchorius citation, see B. F. Huppé, *A Reding of the Canterbury Tales*, pp. 19–20. See also Edith Kern, "The Gardens in the *Decameron Cornice*," *PMLA* 66 (1951): 505–23.

31. "Noi, come voi sapete, domane saranno quindici dì, per dovere alcun diporto pigliare a sostentamento della nostra sanità e della vita, cessando le malinconie e' dolori e l'angosce, le quali per la nostra città continuamente, poi che questo pistolenzioso tempo incominciò, si veggono, uscimmo di Firenze. . . ."

32. ". . . i tre giovani . . . a'loro altri piaceri attesero, e esse, quando tempo lor parve, se ne tornarono alle lor case." I thus find it difficult to accept the view expressed by a number of scholars and summarized by Lucia Marino in *The Decameron 'Cornice,'* p. 74: "He brings his *novellieri* back to the city in the belief that withdrawal effects a refreshment and enrichment of the spirit that is comprehensible as an aim only if the individual will re-instate himself in the social environment most favorable to his full development and happiness." See also Marga Cottino-Jones, "The City/Country Conflict in the *Decameron*," *Studi Boccacceschi* 8 (1974): 147–84.

Al-Manbijī's "Report of the Plague:" a treatise on the Plague of 764-65/1362-64 in the Middle East

Michael Dols

In A.D. 1347 the Black Death was introduced into both the eastern and western Mediterranean. The disease was the same, and it seems to have caused a correspondingly high mortality in both regions. The professional medical perception of the disease was also similar: the doctors based their understanding on Galenic principles that had been modified during the medieval period by Arabic commentaries. Despite these common features, however, most Muslims and Christians interpreted the plague quite differently because of their strong religious orientations. Religion was apparently crucial in determining the contrasting social attitudes toward the calamity. These attitudes largely account for the dissimilar social responses that the disease provoked in Muslim and Christian communities.[1]

The social response of the predominantly Muslim population in the Middle East was guided largely by religious principles that were articulated by the 'ulamā' or religio-legal scholars. These principles were derived from pronouncements or sayings concerning plague that were attributed to the Prophet, known as aḥādīth (sing. ḥadīth). In actuality, many of these pious traditions were formulated after the death of the Prophet; those dealing specifically with plague were created in the following century when plague epidemics afflicted the early Muslim empire.[2] Nevertheless, the traditions held special sanctity for later Muslims and were well-known and easily accessible to religious scholars. In particular, there is evidence that the Prophet's pronouncements on plague were communicated directly to the people by the 'ulamā' during the Black Death and later plague epidemics.

Many of the sayings of the Prophet that dealt with plague are, however, clearly contradictory. Therefore, Muslim scholars debated the issue of plague and composed numerous treatises in order to harmonize the conflicting ideas represented by the pious traditions. Controversy focused primarily on three assertions: (1) a Muslim should not enter or flee from a plague-stricken land; (2) plague is a mercy and a martyrdom from God for a Muslim and a punishment for an infidel; and (3) there is no infection.[3]

The goal of the religious scholars was to arrive at a proper understanding of the divine act of a plague epidemic and to recommend a normative scheme of behavior for the Muslim community. The Arabic *Pestschriften* that have survived in the Middle East are devoted entirely to such religio-legal discussions and deal only peripherally with the historical and medical aspects of the disease.[4] These treatises were written from the mid-fourteenth century to the nineteenth century because the constant recurrence of plague epidemics prompted continued dispute.[5]

A good example of this literature is *Fī Akhbār aṭ-ṭāʿūn (Report of the Plague)* by Muḥammad al-Manbijī. The treatise is important because of its early date and the rarity of contemporary Arabic accounts of plague in the mid-fourteenth century, yet it has not been previously studied. Al-Manbijī composed the work at the end of a plague epidemic in 764–65/1362–64, which was the first major reappearance of plague in Syria after the Black Death. Regarding Muḥammad al-Manbijī, we know only that he was a jurist of the Ḥanbalite school, the most conservative of the four major schools of orthodox Islamic law; the school was particularly influential in Syria and Palestine in the fourteenth century. Al-Manbijī witnessed the Black Death and reportedly died in A.D. 1383.[6]

Our author came from Manbīj in northern Syria, which had suffered severely from Turkoman and, later, Mongol attacks in the thirteenth and early fourteenth centuries.[7] We know from other sources that the town was stricken by the Black Death, and we have a unique report of supernatural phenomena that were observed there and were directly associated with the pandemic. At the time of the Black Death, the tombs of the prophets Mattā and Ḥanẓalah ibn Khuwaylid (the brother of Khadījah) were revealed to the inhabitants. Streams of light shone from the shrines of Shaykh ʿAqīl al-Manbijī and Shaykh Yanbub outside of the city, and the light from them came over the city. Light also came from the tomb of Shaykh ʿAlī and his shrine on the north side of the city. The lights passed from one to another, and they came together and lasted for four nights until the lights blinded the people of Manbīj. The judge of the city saw this, gathered witnesses, and then reported the events

to the provincial capital of Aleppo.[8] These events during the Black
Death are relevant to our treatise because one of the major objec-
tives of al-Manbijī is to refute the religious significance of similar
supernatural events that took place during the subsequent plague
epidemic of 764–65/1362–64.

Al-Manbijī also wrote a second book as a result of still another
plague epidemic that occurred in Syria from Rajab 775 to
Muḥarram 776/December 1373 to June 1374. It is entitled *Tasliyat
ahl al-maṣā'ib (Consolation for Those in Distress)*.[9] In the introduction
to this later work, al-Manbijī tells us that many good and pious
men died in this epidemic, so that he called it the "Plague of the
Best" (*ṭāʿūn al-'akhyār*). The epidemic also destroyed many children,
and it seems that the author lost a son at this time. Following these
introductory remarks, the author mentions his previous work, which
is our primary concern, and says that he had composed it in
765/1364. But because he had not discussed the spiritual meaning
of adversity for plague victims or prescribed the proper conduct
for their survivors in the first book, the second was "devoted to
the consolation of those who are stricken by misfortune of this
world."[10]

The first book of al-Manbijī, *Report of the Plague*, is historically
more important than the second. To repeat, its composition was
prompted by a plague epidemic in Syria that appeared in 764/1362
and lasted until 765/1364. The treatise survives today in a single
seventeenth-century copy in the collection of the National Library
in Cairo; the manuscript is written in Arabic and contains 157 folio
pages.[11] The *Report of the Plague* consists of an introduction and
twenty-two chapters.[12]

At the outset, al-Manbijī clearly states that he has written this
tract because of the "innovation" (*bidʿah*) that had occurred during
the epidemic (fols. 152b–155a). *Bidʿah* has a precise meaning in
Islamic law: it is a belief or practice for which there is no precedent in the time of the Prophet and which is therefore necessarily
wrong.[13] (The closest and least inexact parallel to *bidʿah* in medieval
Europe is the concept of heresy.) Al-Manbijī condemns, therefore,
a number of beliefs and practices that were current during the recent epidemics because he believed that there was no precedent
for them in the Qur'ān, the teaching and example of the Prophet,
or more especially in the lives of the Prophet's companions, for
plague had struck the nascent Muslim community in Syria during
the caliphate of ʿUmar ibn al-Khaṭṭāb (13–23/634–644).[14]

Specifically, al-Manbijī strongly condemns as innovators those who claimed to have seen the Prophet in dreams and complained to him about the plague. Our author calls such claims "heretical and outrageous" and compares them to similar rumors that had circulated during the Black Death.[15] These people had asked the Prophet for special prayers to raise the severe affliction. Al-Manbijī is quite antagonistic, in principle, to the idea that one should seek to revoke what God, in His infinite wisdom, had decreed. Further, al-Manbijī was greatly annoyed at seeing written accounts of these visions and the prayers that the Prophet was said to have supplied circulate among the people. One pious man had told al-Manbijī that he made fifty or sixty copies of the prescribed prayers. Our author said to the man: "The Prophet does not command in sleep what conflicts with wakefulness" (fol. 154a). Nevertheless, copies of such prayers were distributed among the people. Furthermore, al-Manbijī condemns the communal supplications for the lifting of the plague that took place at this time and for the same reason. He asserts that this innovation was introduced during the time of the Black Death; we know that such communal activity did take place in Syria and Egypt during the Black Death.[16] The supplication consisted of fasting and then going out in procession to the desert for communal prayer; it was based on the traditional ritual for rain (*ṣalāt al-istisqāʾ*). Hence, the people, including the notables of the city, assembled and went out en masse to the desert to pray, often accompanying their retreat with loud lamentations. Al-Manbijī describes this penitential ritual and strongly disapproves of it; he observes contemptuously that the plague was lighter before their prayer and greater after it (fol. 155a).

These introductory remarks to our author's treatise alert us to his very conservative attitude toward the subject — the strict reliance on legal precedent for proper beliefs and practices during a plague epidemic — a rigorism which is, in fact, sustained throughout the work.

The subsequent chapters deal at length with the pious traditions regarding plague which we have described. Al-Manbijī argues forcefully in favor of all three principles. On the first point, that a faithful Muslim should not enter or flee from a plague-stricken land, he affirms the prohibition although he recognizes the existence of contradictory traditions and the divergent opinions of other jurists (fols. 186b–200b). According to one tradition, flight from a plague epidemic was analogous to flight from the army. If one is caught in an epidemic, the author recommends prayer, but it should not be for the raising of the disease or for death itself (fols. 165a–168b). Prayer for lifting the epidemic is abhorrent because plague is a blessing from God; at the least, a Muslim should devoutly accept the divine act (fol. 161b–165a).[17]

Therefore, the pious Muslim should suffer an epidemic patiently, trusting in God's will. If one survived the ordeal, the patient endurance of the scourge would eventually be rewarded in the afterlife (fols. 172a–173a). If death came, however, the pious Muslim could expect his reward immediately; his entry into Paradise, like that of the martyrs, was guaranteed. This expectation of the plague victim was based on the second tenet, that plague is a mercy and a martyrdom for the Muslim and a punishment for the infidel. Al-Manbijī fully endorses this belief on the basis of the *aḥādīth* although he recognizes the early controversy over the interpretation of plague, which must have been influenced by contemporary Jewish and Christian views (fols. 168b–172a, 173a–175b). The orthodox view held that the plague-stricken were analogous to the martyrs of Islam because they had been "pierced" by the jinn at God's command, the plague symptoms being held equivalent to the wounds of the martyrs. Therefore, death by plague ideally should be earnestly desired. Al-Manbijī concedes, however, that the disease was also a punishment by God on impious Muslims who committed prohibited acts, such as eating forbidden foods, committing adultery, exacting usury, or consorting with prostitutes (fols. 155a–161b). For the non-Muslim, plague was unquestionably a divine punishment (fols. 168b–172a, 173a–175b). To some extent, this interpretation of plague tried to make sense of the indiscriminate attack of every segment of the population.

Al-Manbijī also endorses the last traditional tenet, that there is no interhuman transmission of plague, for disease comes directly from God. His vehement support for this teaching, even more than for the other two ideas, attests to a popular belief to the contrary. Some Muslims, according to the author, did not visit the sick or accompany the biers of the dead to their graves because of their fear of contamination. He especially attacks the doctors for their belief that plague was infectious although al-Manbijī admits, quite inconsistently, that leprosy, gonorrhea, and scabies are infectious diseases (fols. 224a–231a). In this matter, our author well represents the religious constraint on the physicians who recognized empirically the infectious nature of the disease, especially in a pneumonic plague epidemic.

Despite al-Manbijī's animosity toward the doctors, he uses a number of medical works — both of professional medicine and of "prophetic" or folk medicine — to describe the symptoms of plague. The classical medical works attribute the cause of the disease to a *miasma* or corruption of the air (fols. 183b-186b). However, al-Manbijī rejects this ancient etiology of plague. He asserts that the jinn are the causal agents; the jinn pierce men's bodies with plague-bearing arrows at God's command. Again, the reason for this belief is the author's close adherence to the traditions of the Prophet that profess this supernatural idea (fols. 175b-183b). Similarly, on the authority of the Prophet, al-Manbijī claims that plague would not spread to Mecca and Medina, regardless of the fact that the Black Death had been quite destructive in Mecca (fols. 178a, 200b-201b).

Furthermore, al-Manbijī relates that during the Black Death the doctors had been very ineffectual in healing the sick and the number of physicians had been seriously diminished (fols. 204b-205a) — but even more ignorant and misleading than the doctors, according to our author, were the diviners and fortune-tellers during the epidemic of 764-65/1362-64. Al-Manbijī is particularly hostile toward astrologers, who seem to have been very popular (fols. 203b-207b). A pious Muslim should not believe in augury or omens but should trust in God entirely (fol. 224a).

As do the authors of other plague treatises in the Middle East, al-Manbijī discusses the seriousness of the disease (fols. 208b-210b), the Arabic terminology for plague (fols. 202a-203b),[18] and the chronology of plague epidemics in the Islamic era (fols. 210b-223b). In al-Manbijī's chronicle of epidemics, he alleges that plague was unknown to the Arabs before the advent of Islam (fols. 201b-202a), but that it repeatedly attacked the early Muslim empire in the Middle East; this history is based primarily on the accounts of al-Madā-'inī (d. 225/840), al-Aṣmaʿī through the works of Ibn Qutaybah (d. 276/889), and Ibn Abī d-Dunyā (d. 281/894). Between the Umayyad Period and the advent of the Black Death, al-Manbijī lists epidemics in Egypt in 445/1053-54 and Constantinople in 447/1055-56 on the authority of Ibn Buṭlān (d. 458/1066);[19] a serious epidemic in central Asia in 449/1057 that spread to the Middle East; epidemics in Egypt in 455/1063, Damascus in 469/1076-77, and Iraq in 478/1085; and a plague named after Ibn

Hubayrah, a famous 'Abbāsid *wazīr* and jurist of Baghdad, who is reported to have died in the epidemic of 560/1165.[20] Incidentally, concerning the epidemic that struck Damascus in 469/1076–77, al-Manbijī tells us the story of a woman who saw a large number of rats in the city; she bought some cats to kill the rodents and then sold cats to others at a considerable profit. To my knowledge, this is the *only* instance in the Arabic historical literature where rats are closely associated with a plague epidemic. In view of our modern understanding of plague pathology, it is extraordinary that rodent mortality is never mentioned in the sources.

Concerning the Black Death in the Middle East — about which we would like to know a great deal more — al-Manbijī is unfortunately reticent. Yet he is our only source for the fact that the pandemic was called by some the "Plague of 'Amwās," which was the name of the first great plague epidemic in Islamic history.[21] Furthermore, he relates that the Black Death and the plague of 764–65/1362–64 were common to Syria, Egypt, and Iraq as well as the lands of the infidel, and that both caused a great mortality. Between these two epidemics, al-Manbijī says that there was a serious epidemic of plague in Egypt in 761/1360, when the commodities demanded by the plague-stricken, especially quince, became very costly.

This history of epidemics is important because of its early date. Before studying this manuscript, this author believed that the first full enumeration of epidemics, including plague, written after the Black Death was that of Ibn Abī Ḥajalah; his treatise was composed sometime between 764/1362 and his death in the plague epidemic of 776/1375.[22] Al-Manbijī's chronology, however, was written in 765/1363–64, apparently independently of Ibn Abī Ḥajalah's work. Moreover, al-Manbijī's *Report of the Plague* appears to be the earliest example of the plague treatise as a literary genre that was developed exclusively in the Middle East after the Black Death. Al-Manbijī's work lacks only the cursory medical prescriptions for plague victims that are characteristic of the later treatises. The precedence of al-Manbijī's tract and its relationship to Ibn Abī Ḥajalah's treatise remains to be firmly established; the latter, however, was far more influential while the former is rarely mentioned in the later treatises.[23]

In conclusion, the treatise of al-Manbijī initiates or, at least, contributes to a new tradition of systematic legal discourse on the Prophetic pronouncements regarding plague.[24] His work has special importance because we have very few contemporary sources for the history of the Black Death and its immediate recurrences in the Middle East. The treatise supplies us with some new information as well as confirming our general understanding of the social consequences of the Black Death in this region. It does not, however, contain detailed information about the history of al-Manbijī's city during either the Black Death or the epidemic of 764–65/1362–64. Like the other treatise writers, al-Manbijī was a religious scholar whose concern was not historical, although his work does afford glimpses of contemporary events.

Al-Manbijī's primary concern was the elucidation and propagation of Islamic law, which should guide the lives of faithful Muslims.[25] In this manner, al-Manbijī represents the communal leadership of the *ulamā'*, who set the boundaries to conflicting ideas about plague and communal activities. In his judgment the law had been seriously misunderstood or disregarded during the recent epidemics.

Al-Manbijī's exposition of the law is not persuasive; it is poorly organized and does not resolve satisfactorily the numerous difficulties caused by the conflicting traditions. In the light of the other later plague treatises, the author's rigid adherence to the pious traditions is striking, the most remarkable example of his orthodoxy being his hostility toward medicine and divination. In general, al-Manbijī presents a very conservative viewpoint that was influential in determining social attitudes. Such a point of view helps us to explain the relatively pacific reaction of Muslim society to plague epidemics. Paradoxically, the treatise demonstrates by its conservatism the range of possible interpretations that were accessible to Muslims in the mid-fourteenth century and, by its criticism of communal behavior, attests to the existence of differing beliefs and practices.

notes

1. For a comparison of Muslim and Christian responses to the Black Death, see Dols, *The Black Death in the Middle East* (Princeton, 1977), pp. 284–301.

2. Miklos Muranyi, *Die Prophetengenossen in der Frühislamischen Geschichte,* Bonner Orientalistische Studien, n.s. 28 (Bonn, 1973), pp. 114–15. The author asserts that traditions concerning plague were prompted by the outbreaks of plague in Kūfah toward the end of the first century A.H. and originated in the circle of the family of Sa'd ibn Abī Waqqās.

3. In my discussion of the prohibition of the idea of infection, I have interpreted "infection" ('adwā) in the Arabic texts in a broad sense to mean both contagion and infection. In modern medical terminology, this is quite unacceptable. "Contagion" means the transmission of the disease by an agent while "infection" implies the lack of such an agent and the communication of the bacilli directly. With regard to plague, the distinction is an important one; bubonic plague is contagious, whereas pneumonic plague is infectious. While this distinction is helpful in understanding the historical phenomenon of the Black Death, no such distinction was made in the medieval treatises on plague. In the present context, a better translation might be: there is no transmissibility of disease; see the discussion of Manfred Ullmann, *Islamic Medicine* (Edinburgh, 1978), pp. 86–96.

4. For a more detailed discussion of the religious principles and a survey of the *Pestschriften,* see Dols, *The Black Death in the Middle East,* pp. 109–21, 291–93, and Appendix 3.

5. See Dols, "The Second Plague Pandemic and Its Recurrences in the Middle East: 1347-1894," *The Journal of the Economic and Social History of the Orient* 22 (1978): 162–89; Boaz Shoshan, "Notes sur les epidemics de peste en Egypti," *Annales de Démographie Historique* (1981): 387–404.

6. Sami K. Hamarneh, *History of Arabic Medicine and Pharmacy* (Cairo, 1967), pt. 1, pp. 60–61; pt. 2, pp. 22–23.

7. "Manbidj" (E. Honigmann) in *The Encyclopaedia of Islam* (Leiden-London, 1913–34).

8. Ibn al-Wardī, *Tatimmat al-mukhtaṣar* (Cairo, A. H. 1285), vol. 2, pp. 353–54; see Dols, *The Black Death in the Middle East,* pp. 62, 252–53.

9. Cairo, 1929. See Dols, *The Black Death in the Middle East,* pp. 242n, 328; Carl Brockelmann, *Geschichte der arabischen Literatur* (Leiden, 1945–49), 2:76; *Supplement* (Leiden, 1937–42), 2:82.

10. Muḥammad al-Manbijī, *Tasliyat al-maṣāʾib* (Cairo, 1929), pp. 3–4, 201.

11. Dār al-Kutub al-Miṣrīyah MS no. 16 ṭibb Halīm, fols. 152a–231a.

12. While the subject matter has been treated thematically in my discussion of the work, it may be helpful for future investigators to list the chapter headings: (1) the reasons for the occurence of plague (155a–161b); (2) the abhorrence of prayer for the lifting of plague (161b–165a); (3) the desirabili-

ty of prayer at the time of plague (165a–168b); (4) the desirability of martyrdom (168b–171b); (5) plague is a martyrdom for Muslims but not for others (171b–172a); (6) patience during plague (172a–173a); (7) plague is a mercy for the community (173a–175b); (8) the prayer of the Prophet during plague (175b–180b); (9) plague is the piercing of our enemies by the jinn (180b–182b); (10) the harmonization of the words of the Prophet (182a–183b); (11) description of plague (183b–186b); (12) the prohibition on entering or fleeing a plague-stricken area (186b–192a); (13) the prohibition on fleeing plague (192a–199a); (14) differences among scholars on the ban (199a–200b); (15) plague does not enter Mecca and Medina (200b–201b); (16) whether the pre-Islamic Arabs knew plague or not (201b–202a); (17) the meaning of *ṭāʿūn* and *wabāʾ* (202a–203b); (18) rebuttal to the astrologers (203b–207b); (19) what our ancestors did in a plague epidemic (207b–208b); (20) whether plague was a fatal disease (208b–210b); (21) chronicle of plagues in the Islamic era (210b–224a); and (22) abhorrence of infection and omens (224a–231a).

13. "Bidʿa" (J. Robson) in *The Encyclopaedia of Islam,* new ed. (Leiden-London, 1960 –).

14. See Dols, "Plague in Early Islamic History," *Journal of the American Oriental Society* 94 (1974): 371–83, and Dols, *The Black Death in the Middle East,* pp. 13–35; Lawrence Conrad, "The Plague in the Early Medieval Near East," Diss., Princeton University, 1981, pp. 120–246.

15. See Dols, *The Black Death in the Middle East,* pp. 120, 127, 251–52.

16. Ibid., pp. 120, 246–52.

17. Parenthetically, there is a marginal note in the manuscript alongside this discussion that is significant: a description of communal prayer in Cairo during the plague epidemic of 769/1367–68. The information is valuable because we have practically no other evidence for this epidemic (fols. 161b–165a).

18. On Arabic terminology, see Dols, *The Black Death in the Middle East,* App. 2; for corrections and refinements, see Lawrence Conrad, *"Ṭāʿūn* and *Wabāʾ*: Conceptions of Plague and Pestilence in Early Islam," *Journal of the Economic and Social History of the Orient* (in press).

19. *Cf.* Ibn Abī Uṣaybiʿah *ʿUyūn al-anbāʾ*, ed. A. Müller, vol. 1 (Cairo, 1882), p. 242.

20. "Ibn Hubayra" (G. Makdisi) in *The Encyclopaedia of Islam*, new ed.

21. Concerning ʿAmwās, see Dols, *The Black Death in the Middle East,* p. 21 and passim; for Arabic terminology of the Black Death, see ibid., p. 5, n. 5.

22. *Dafʿ an-niqmah fī ṣ-ṣalāt ʿalā nabī r-raḥmān,* Escorial MS no. 1772, fols. 1a–87b; for the history of epidemics, see fols. 59b–76b.

23. Lawrence Conrad, "Arabic Plague Chronologies and Treatises: Social and Historical Factors in the Formation of a Literary Genre," *Studia Islamica* 54(1981): 51–93, claims that Ibn Abī Ḥajalah's treatise is the earliest of this literature.

24. Al-Manbijī's stance toward many of the issues closely resembles that

of Ibn Ḥajar al-'Asqalānī in his later and better known plague treatise; see Dols, *The Black Death in the Middle East,* p. 110 and passim, and Jacqueline Sublet, "La Peste prise aux rêts de la jurisprudence: Le Traité d'Ibn Ḥajar al-'Asqalānī sur la peste," *Studia Islamica* 33 (1971): 141–49.

25. Based on the treatise of Ibn Abī Ḥajalah and especially his plague chronology, Conrad ("Arabic Plague Chronologies and Treatises") contends that the major theme of the plague tracts was the consolation of the endangered or aggrieved reader during a plague epidemic. This is clearly the purpose of al-Manbijī's *Tasliyat* but not of the present work. It seems very misleading, therefore, to suggest such a purpose for the entire genre of plague treatises.

the Black Death and Western European Eschatological mentalities

Robert E. Lerner

As there is a "Richter scale" for measuring earthquakes, so there is now a "Foster scale" for measuring disasters. Harold D. Foster, a Canadian geographer, has maintained that disasters ought not to be ranked solely by their toll in lives but also by the physical damage and emotional stress they create. By these standards the Black Death of 1347 to 1350 falls two-tenths of a point short of being the worst disaster in history: on the Foster scale, World War II (11.1) ranks first, the Black Death (10.9) second, and World War I (10.5) third.[1]

Without stopping to quibble about the two-tenths of a point, or to ask whether one can calibrate emotional stress so finely, we might agree that the Black Death was one of the worst disasters on record. Among the numerous vivid illustrations of the horror are a German chronicler's image of ships floating with dead crews aimlessly on the seas and an Italian chronicler's offhand hyperbole that "there was not a dog left pissing on the wall."[2] Granted that the disaster was enormous, the question to be asked here is, how was it placed within the framework of eschatological thought? At a time when people believed seriously in the end of the world and the Last Judgment, how did they place the onslaught of the greatest disaster yet known within their conception of the history of salvation?

Obviously, even during the greatest of disasters, not everybody reacts in the same way. Robert Benchley once remarked that in every news photo of epoch-making events there always seems to be a man in a derby hat looking in the opposite direction from the action: on Bloody Sunday in St. Petersburg or assassination day in Sarajevo, a "Johnny-on-the-spot" is always looking up at a clock, picking his teeth, or waving insouciantly at the camera. Quite apart from those who lived in parts of Europe where the Black Death did not strike, there were probably some people in 1348 or 1349 who went about their business or pleasure in the eye of the storm. They may have given no thought to the end of the world or the events that might precede it and would have waved at the camera had there been one to wave at. Hence, I do not mean to argue that everyone in Europe, when confronted by the plague, thought about the history of salvation. (It would be good to know how many did and how many did not, but unfortunately we never can.) What I do mean to argue is that the onslaught of disaster did lead many to wonder about how it fit into God's plan, and the ways in which they did so are of considerable interest to the cultural historian.

Indisputably, many in Western Europe took the plague to be an eschatological sign. The Arabic chronicler as-Sulūk reported that Christians on Cyprus who experienced the Black Death "feared that it was the end of the world."[3] As-Sulūk probably misunderstood their fear somewhat, because no medieval Christian believed that the world would end without certain culminating events — such as the reign of Antichrist — preceding the Last Judgment. But, certainly, many thought that the Black Death signaled God's displeasure and in some way presaged the End. A Franciscan chronicler of Lübeck, for example, wrote that the Black Death was a divine punishment for human evil and a sign of the last days, qualifying this assessment with the assurance that exactly when those days would come God alone knew. Similarly, the Swiss Franciscan, John of Winterthur, claimed that a great earthquake of 1348 and the plague (which had not yet hit his own region) were antecedents of the terrible disasters that the Lord had warned would come before his Second Coming (Matthew 24:7; Luke 21:11).[4]

Although helpful to start with, such statements not only leave open the question of how long it would be before the End would arrive — respecting Christ's injunction in Acts 1:7 that "it is not for you to know the times or the seasons which the Father hath put in his own power" — but also say nothing about what might happen between the time of the plague and the Last Judgment. Yet people surely speculated on just that point. What might their thoughts have been?

Remarkably little research has been done on this subject, perhaps because scholars have been unaware of evidence that would help

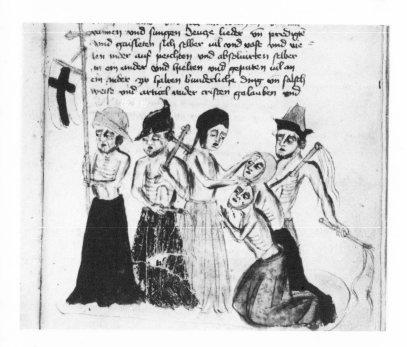

Fig. 1: A flagellant procession at the time of the Black Death. Illustration taken from the *Konstanzer*, third quarter of the fifteenth century, Bavaria; Munich, Bayerische Staatsbibliothek, MS Cgm 426, f. 42v.

them treat it. Hitherto, the only approach has been through the sensational — the macabre processions of the flagellants. In the nineteenth century Herman Haupt connected the flagellant processions with eschatological prophecies and maintained that "the flagellants felt called upon to prepare the way for the coming kingdom of God." Dilating on this theme, Norman Cohn has written that the German flagellants of 1349 were "eschatologically inspired hordes" whose activities "ended as a militant and bloody pursuit of the Millennium." Like Cohn, Philip Ziegler stated in a popular book on the Black Death that the German flagellants conceived of their movement ending "only with the redemption of Christendom and the arrival of the Millenium [*sic*]." Similarly, the East German scholar Martin Erbstösser, limiting his argument to the flagellants of Thuringia and Franconia (who he believed were more radical than the others), argued that the flagellants "felt themselves to be the proclaimers of a new time, that of the preparation for the end of the world."[5]

The flagellants, then, it is commonly assumed, were millenarians. I also think it likely that they were, but I must concede with Richard A. Kieckhefer that the assumption is based on very slender evidence. Putting aside the later "cryptoflagellants," whose millenarianism is not in doubt, only two sources speak in any way of flagellant millenarianism, and neither of these presents incontrovertible proof.[6] The first and somewhat more detailed of these sources is an increasingly familiar friend of the heresiologist known as the Breslau manuscript. The anonymous author of a theological *questio* in this fifteenth-century manuscript attributed to the flagellants an eschatological song, which stated that in seventeen years after 1349, after many tribulations, the religious orders, particularly the mendicants, would expire, to be replaced by a new one. After that, the old orders would be restored "with great glory" and then the world would end.[7]

One problem with this report is chronological, for the theological *questio* postdates the appearance of the Hussites in the early fifteenth century. As Kieckhefer has noted, even if the author thought he was writing about the flagellants of 1349, he may have confused their ideas with those of the cryptoflagellants or attributed to them a song that they had not sung.[8] That may be hypercritical: perhaps the flagellants of 1349 did sing about great changes coming within seventeen years. But the song in question still does not show them to be the eschatological radicals portrayed by Cohn, Ziegler, and Erbstösser. Cohn in particular appears to have distorted the evidence by interpreting the song as, "of course, . . . a prophecy in the Joachite tradition." According to him, "it is certain that when [the] flagellants talked of a new monastic order of unique holiness they were referring to themselves alone."[9] But, in fact, the flagellants in the song never say this. Moreover, the text does not pose a clear opposition between the old orders and the new one—that is, a "Joachite" opposition between an old and a new dispensation— but instead foretells the ultimate glorious restoration of the old orders. In short, the passage says nothing about a revolutionary role for the flagellants; it merely foresees a time of tribulations followed by one of "great glory" before the End.

The other source that seems to contain some evidence of flagellant eschatological hopes is the "heavenly letter" reportedly read aloud during a flagellant sermon in Strassburg. This text, supposedly brought to earth by an angel, tells of Christ's anger with rampant impiety, warns of great punishments, and calls for reform and penance. But it also promises that, if men were to change their ways, Christ's anger would be assuaged and a time of blessedness and fruitfulness for the earth would ensue.[10] Aside from the vagueness of this promise, the difficulty with the passage for assessing flagellant views is that it did not originate with the flagellants. The heavenly letter was a text put forward repeatedly in different versions throughout the Middle Ages, and the part in question is known to have been formulated by about 1200 at the latest.[11] If the flagellants paid any particular attention to it, how central it was to their own beliefs is still impossible to know.

Cohn called the heavenly letter the "manifesto of the flagellant movement." Whether or not there is any truth in this designation, the letter was certainly not a manifesto for revolutionary millenarian action, for the clear and simple message of the text read in its entirety is the call to "repent and be saved."[12] Whatever the flagellants' ideas about the future, there is little question that the driving motivation behind their processions was not to "pursue the millennium" but to do penance in the hope of appeasing God's wrath and thereby warding off the plague. If the flagellants were millenarians (and, as I said, I think they were), they were to that degree not unusual but typical of their age. In my view, most who thought about the significance of the plague were millenarians or chiliasts. Inasmuch as this may be controversial, the rest of this essay will be devoted to explaining and supporting my contention.

Although the word "chiliasm" has taken on for some the connotation of being more extreme than millenarianism, I consider the two words to be synonymous because both have the same etymology — coming respectively from the Greek and Latin for one thousand. In what follows, I use chiliasm instead of millenarianism simply because it is less cumbersome. Along with most scholars, I do not limit chiliasm to belief in a literal thousand-year kingdom ruled over by Christ but define the term more broadly to mean the expectation of imminent, supernaturally inspired, radical betterment on earth before the Last Judgment. Where I differ from some scholars is in my belief that chiliasm does not have to be oriented toward revolutionary action, although it certainly can be. Rather, it can also encourage perseverance in the face of persecution and bring hope in the face of trials.[13]

There were two main varieties of chiliasm in the Middle Ages: the "post-Antichrist" and the "pre-Antichrist" strains.[14] The former

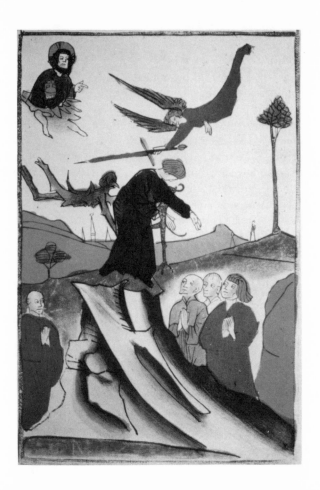

Fig. 2: Antichrist prepares for his false ascension and Archangel Michael descends to smite him. Reproduced from *Buch von dem Entkrist*, colored woodcuts, mid-fifteenth century. (Photograph provided by Professor Gerald Strauss, Indiana University.)

was more grounded in traditional biblical exegesis than the latter and, therefore, was more often expressed in formal treatises by identifiable writers. Building upon agreement in the standard early medieval biblical commentaries of St. Jerome on Daniel 12:11–12, the Venerable Bede on Revelation 8:1, and Haimo of Auxerre on the Pauline epistles (I Thessalonians 5:3 and II Thessalonians 2:8) that there would be a period of intermission on earth between the demise of Antichrist and the Last Judgment, numerous twelfth-century writers independently expressed varieties of post-Antichrist chiliasm. Whereas the early medieval authorities abhorred chiliasm and only allowed the idea of a final time on earth because Scrip-

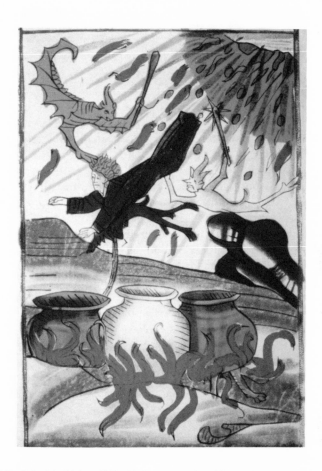

Fig. 3: Devils lead Antichrist to Hell, with the representation of fire and brime stone. Reproduced from *Buch von dem Entkrist*, colored woodcuts, mid-fifteenth century. (Photograph provided by Professor Gerald Strauss, Indiana University.)

ture seemed to offer no alternative, such thoroughly orthodox twelfth-century commentators as Honorius Augustodunensis, Otto of Freising, Hildegard of Bingen, Gerhoch of Reichersberg, and the anonymous author of the *Glossa ordinaria* on Daniel welcomed the idea of a final time after Antichrist and made it serve variously for the "refreshment of the saints," the conversion of the heathen and the Jews, and the reformation and purification of the Church. In Gerhoch of Reichersberg's view, the time after Antichrist would be one of "great joy for the people of God."

The theory of a wondrous time on earth after the death of Antichrist was brought to its first full flowering at the end of the twelfth century in the luxuriantly fertile prophetic writings of the Calabrian abbot, Joachim of Fiore. Joachim granted the last time the dignity of being a full historical age by making it serve concurrently as the seventh age of the Church, the seventh age of the world, and the third "status" of historical progress typified by the unfolding of the Trinity. In addition, Joachim was the first medieval exegete to read the most explicitly chiliastic passage in the Bible, the prediction of the reign of the saints with Christ on earth in Revelation 20, as alluding to the time after Antichrist. Finally, Joachim broadened the positive conception of the final time still wider than did other twelfth-century writers: for him it would be marked not just by profound peace and the conversion of unbelievers but also by the highest possible levels of ecclesiastical organization and human spiritual illumination short of Paradise.

Owing to its firm anchoring in standard biblical exegesis and to the gathering momentum of its elaborations, the idea of a wondrous time on earth after Antichrist became a virtually unquestioned assumption of Western eschatological theology from 1200 until the end of the Middle Ages. To take only one example, a "best-selling" theological handbook designed as a convenient reference work for the use of clerics, Hugh Ripelin's *Compendium theologicae veritatis* (ca. 1265), stated as a certainty that "after Antichrist's death the Lord will not come immediately to judgment" but, rather, that there would be a time of "refreshment of the saints" when "the Jews will be converted to the faith and the Holy Church will peacefully conquer everything up to the ends of the earth." Like several other exponents of post-Antichrist chiliasm, Hugh Ripelin was probably not influenced by Joachim of Fiore. Undoubtedly, many others were. But as long as they affirmed, as almost all did, that the dispensation of the last age would be a renewal and amplification of the Christian dispensation announced in the Gospels rather than a supercession of it, they were not stating anything controversial.

With theologians agreeing that there would be good times on earth after Antichrist, anyone in the mid-fourteenth century who assumed that Antichrist's open reign would be preceded by heralding disasters could easily incorporate the Black Death into a chiliastic script. Such a script, in fact, exists in John of Rupescissa's still unpublished *Liber secretorum eventuum*, completed in November 1349.[15] Rupescissa, a Franciscan visionary who was then being held in a papal prison in Avignon because of his attacks on the Franciscan and ecclesiastical hierarchies, predicted that Antichrist would

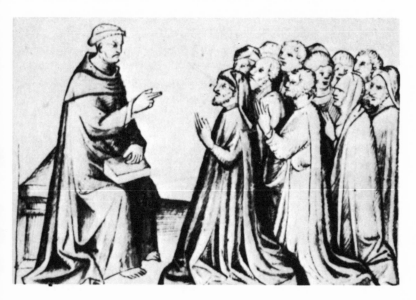

Fig. 4: The triumph of the "holy people of God" on earth after the death of Antichrist. A conception descending from Rupescissa in Telephorus, *Libellus* . . . , written toward the end of the fourteenth century. The illumination is reproduced from Munich, Bayerische Staatsbibliothek, MS Clm 313, f. 38v, executed shortly after 1431 in or around Salzburg.

triumph and reign openly for three and a half years before 1370 and that, before then, numerous chastisements would precede his arrival. First among these was the famine and plague Rupescissa dated to 1347, and second was the piling up of cadavers of the year 1348.[16] Famine and plague would be followed by earthquakes and other disasters, culminating in the reign of Antichrist. But in 1370 Christ would slay Antichrist and ordain a literal millennium — one thousand years of earthly blessedness before the End. During the forty-five years between 1370 and 1415, there would still be wars resulting in the transference of the Roman Empire to Jerusalem, but then would come a millennium of the greatest possible earthly perfection when men would beat their swords into plowshares and live under the fullness of the Holy Spirit in unprecedented peace and justice. Only toward the end of the millennium would charity begin to grow cold until Gog and Magog would arrive around 2370, presaging the Last Judgment and the end of the world.

Rupescissa's view of the future was obviously shaped by

knowledge of post-Antichrist chiliasm in its Joachite cast, but autobiographical passages in his writings display how he was moved to his own formulation of it by personal stress. In December 1344, he had been arrested without any warning by order of the Franciscan Provincial of Aquitaine and dragged from his native convent of Aurillac to imprisonment in the convent of Figeac, where he was held in particularly noisome quarters. In February 1345, he broke his leg and was forced two or three times onto a device to set it, which made him suffer, according to his account, the torments of the martyrs. Then he was left lying on a cot virtually without attendance for three and a half months while so many maggots crawled in his festering wound that they could be gathered by the handful. By the summer Rupescissa had recovered, but he still was in chains, surrounded by stench, and, hence, spent his days in tears, vigils, and prayers, seeking to understand why he had been made to suffer so terribly. Then, all of a sudden, in late July (one can imagine the heat), while he was standing in prayer, he was granted a miraculous flash of insight into the entire course of the present and future. This revelation made it clear that Antichrist would soon triumph and that Rupescissa was suffering as a "witness" against Antichristian forces but that there would soon be millennial rewards for the witnesses and martyrs after Antichrist's destruction.[17]

Rupescissa'a revelation of July 1345 could not have included foreknowledge of the Black Death, but he soon learned of that horror very personally. In 1348 he became infected with the plague himself while he was imprisoned in another miserable Franciscan confinement, this time at Rieux, south of Toulouse.[18] Rupescissa escaped with his life but again suffered greatly and saw, whether in reality or delirium, swarms of terrible flies that seemed like apocalyptic locusts.[19] Thus, not surprisingly, he built the plague into his understanding of present and future between 1348 and 1349. God was punishing humanity in numerous ways that would culminate in Antichrist's imminent triumph, but proper understanding of the future offered a beacon of hope and a guide for enduring through tribulation.

Although Rupescissa's *Liber secretorum eventuum* was meant only for the private reference of Cardinal Guillaume Court, who was then investigating the imprisoned prophet's orthodoxy, the work traveled quickly beyond Avignon and had a very wide circulation. Five surviving Latin copies and one complete Catalan translation

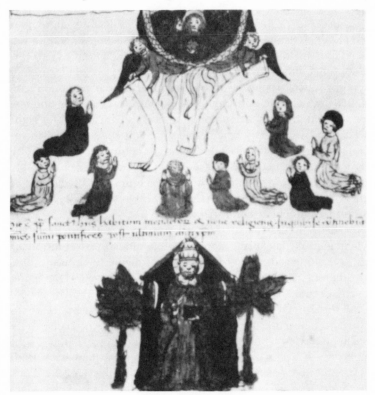

Fig. 5: The Holy Spirit raining down on the elect after the death of Antichrist, with a "holy pope" below, from Telesphorus, *Libellus.* . . . This copy was made in 1469 in the Venetian monastery of St. Cyprian; Venice, Biblioteca Marciana, MS Lat. Cl. III, 177 (2176), f. 35r. (Photograph provided by Professor E. Kaske, Cornell University.)

are only partial testimonies to its popularity, for the *Liber* became known very rapidly to chroniclers and was frequently excerpted or abbreviated.[20] Quite clearly, it struck upon some responsive chords.

As opposed to post-Antichrist chiliasm, the pre-Antichrist variety had virtually no biblical underpinning and, therefore, was seldom espoused openly by theologians. Nonetheless, it appears to have been more "popular" than the post-Antichrist form, in the sense both of having been expressed more frequently and of having wider currency among nonliterate classes. Ever since the eleventh century, the view that a last great emperor would inaugurate wondrous times on earth before the appearance of Antichrist had en-

joyed great favor in Western Europe as a result of its circulation
first in the extremely popular prophecies of Pseudo-Methodius and
the "Tiburtine Sibyl" and then in numerous adaptations and im-
itations that often introduced kings or popes in place of the original
emperor. Such prophecies were naturally reformulated and recir-
culated by dynastic and papal propagandists, and they unquestionably found resonance among the masses who longed for right
order to be installed by epic heroes. Pre-Antichrist chiliastic prophecies were very often pseudonymous or anonymous, but that by
no means impeded their circulation.[21] Indeed, considerable
evidence, most of which has hitherto been unstudied, shows that
different contemporaries independently fitted the Black Death into the pre-Antichrist chiliastic scheme.

In their discussions of the background for alleged flagellant
eschatological radicalism, Haupt, Cohn, and Erbstösser introduced two examples of the second variety of medieval chiliasm, but,
for different reasons, these are the least conclusive.[22] One is the
oft-cited report by John of Winterthur that around 1348 people
"of all sorts" in Germany said that the emperor Frederick II would
return to persecute the clergy, reform the Church, redistribute
wealth, and reign in justice before resigning his crown on the Mount
of Olives. As feverishly intense as these expressions may have been,
they cannot be associated directly with the incidence of the Black
Death because, as Haupt and others have hesitated to acknowledge,
they were current in Germany before the plague struck.[23]

The second example was connected with the Black Death, but,
unfortunately, it survives in a form that is barely usable. According to the Würzburg chronicler Michael de Leone, a certain "great
astrologer" "predicted" for 1348 the coming of a "great dearth and
pestilence." No doubt this was prediction after the fact; Michael
himself clearly recognized the pestilence as the Black Death, because
in 1349 he commented that such was "already coming true in many
parts of Lombardy."[24] The astrologer also "predicted" many other
events, but there are doubts about whether Michael de Leone
reported them in correct order or whether he abbreviated them excessively. For example, the list of predictions contains a brief statement that the "tyrannous king of France would fall with all of his
barons"; this sounds very much like a prophecy after the fact of
Philip VI's defeat at Crécy in 1346, but that would make it two
years off the mark and, coming after the Black Death, not in proper order. Thus, it is difficult to know how to order the astrologer's

predictions of disasters that had apparently not yet come, such as an infestation of insects and poisonous animals, or exactly how to interpret his predictions of the coming of "a single lord" and the "exaltation of the Roman Empire." As best as can be told, however, the last two predictions appear to have been expressions of the perennial imperial prophecies that foretold the coming of a great messianic ruler before the time of Antichrist.[25]

Both John of Winterthur and Michael de Leone were chroniclers who told of prophecies at second hand. Scholarly reliance on them has been typical of a general reliance on chronicle sources as evidence for medieval eschatological ideas. But numerous prophecies that circulated independently of the chronicles help bring us much closer to the original nature and quality of medieval popular eschatology. Just as John of Rupescissa's unpublished *Liber secretorum eventuum* shows how the Black Death was fitted into the post-Antichrist pattern of chiliasm, so several other unnoticed prophecies reveal how the epidemic was fitted into the pre-Antichrist pattern.

The most detailed example is the neglected prophecy of an obscure Frenchman, John of Bassigny.[26] All we know about this prophet, other than that Bassigny was a small territory in Champagne, comes from the text of his prophecy — and that may not be too trustworthy. John claimed to have derived his knowledge of future events not just from studying Holy Scripture and the writings of the prophets, poets, and many learned authorities but also from conversations he held with a Syrian and a "Chaldean" in 1341 while he was traveling in the Holy Land. But this account may not be reliable, because the Eastern place names he gave appear to be bogus.[27] John also claimed to be predicting events from 1343 onward, but his "prophecies" for the years up to about 1361 were clearly made from a knowledge of events that had already occurred.[28]

According to John of Bassigny, a terrible time of trials for the world would begin in 1344 with the onset of a devasting plague.[29] This was certainly the Black Death, because John described it tellingly as a "general mortality and pest" that would carry off more than half of the population.[30] Most likely he dated its onset three years earlier than the time it first appeared in the West because he was attributing his "prophetic" information to Easterners. John must have assumed that the plague moved from east to west and had no way of knowing when it might have begun in the East. But to leave no doubt in his readers' minds that he was alluding to the Great Plague, he went on to say that it would last for "45 months or more," thereby specifying the actual time of the Black Death's visitation.

In the wake of the plague would follow a succession of horrendous chastisements. Among other things, in 1346, "or a little earlier or later" (a studied vagueness), a great "prince and king of all of the West" would be miserably chased and defeated in battle, and almost all of his knights would be killed—surely a prophecy after the event of the French defeat at Crécy. Similarly, John's "prediction" that "around 1356" the king of France would be captured by his enemies was a prophecy after the event of John the Good's capture by the English at Poitiers. John "predicted" still worse disasters for France for 1358 and 1359, the actual period of the *Jacquerie*, the revolt of Étienne Marcel, and the ravaging of France by the English. Starting around 1361 or 1362 John introduced real prophecy, predicting, for example, the destruction of Paris before 1362.[31] After that, the Church would be terribly persecuted, and the elements would rage.

So far, all was bad, but John was no unmitigated pessimist. A coming young hero (perhaps meaning the future Charles V) would assume the French crown and dominate the world. He would aid the Irish and Scots in invading England and in annihilating the "sons of Brutus" so that there would thereafter be no memory of them. A holy pope would be crowned by angels and bring the Church back to its pristine state of apostolic sanctity. He would go preaching barefoot everywhere and convert the infidels. Then he would ordain a messianic ruler from the "most noble" French line as emperor, and the two would reform and bring peace to the whole world. Under their sway, there would be "one law, one life, and one faith," and all men would be of one spirit and love each other. This time of peace would last for "many years," but then men would return to evil, and times would grow worse until the coming of Antichrist.[32]

John of Bassigny's prophecy circulated quickly—one copy reached northern England a few years after it was written[33]—and must have satisfied a deep need for comprehending the present within the terms of the future. The one drawback to using it as a source for appraising eschatological reactions to the Black Death is that it was not written under the most immediate impact of the plague, at least not at the time of the first occurrence. But another prophetic text, almost entirely neglected by scholarship, dates from the terrible plague year of 1349 itself.

The Carmelite William of Blofield sent a report of "rumors" from "Roman parts" to an unnamed friar in the Dominican convent of Norwich in 1349. According to these rumors, Antichrist was already ten years old and a boy of incomparable beauty and learning. But another boy who lived "beyond the Tartars" and was instructed in Christianity was already twelve years old. He would destroy "the perfidy of the Saracens," become the greatest among Christians, and rule as pope and emperor. His empire, however, would quickly come to an end by violence and thereafter would arise unprecedented "revolutions" throughout the world, out of which would emerge a "good and just pope" who would create cardinals who feared the Lord. In this pope's time there would be the greatest peace, but afterward Antichrist would reign openly. William of Blofield dismissed these rumors as fictitious, but he was nonetheless sufficiently interested in them to communicate them to a Dominican friend, who in turn preserved them at Norwich. Whatever William thought, his report is evidence that speculations about Christian triumph and wondrous times before Antichrist circulated in Italy during the time of the plague.[34]

Still more evidence shows that similar speculations were circulating very widely at the same time throughout Western Europe. In the Middle Ages prophecies did not always have to be invented to fit new situations; old ones could be resurrected with new dates. One that was resurrected to fit the Black Death was a text beginning "the high Cedar of Lebanon will be felled," which circulated in various forms throughout Europe from about 1240 until deep into the seventeenth century and lay at hand during the plague years for someone to revive for the edification of himself and others. The version of the "Cedar of Lebanon" prophecy he used began by reporting that in 1287 a Cistercian monk in Syrian Tripoli had seen a hand writing a prophetic message during mass on the corporal cloth over the altar. The message foretold that Tripoli and Acre would soon fall and that worse disasters would follow: a "people without a head" would come, the "Ship of Peter" would be tossed in the waves, and battles, famines, and plagues would strike everywhere. Then two great rulers, one from the East and the other from the West, would conquer the world and bring peace and "abundance of fruit" for fifteen years. Thereafter would follow a successful crusade, the city of Jerusalem would be "glorified," and the Holy Sepulchre would be visited by all. But in this tranquillity "news would be heard of Antichrist."[35]

The vision of the Cistercian monk was certainly fictitious; much of it was plagiarized from a prophecy of about 1240, and there was not even any Cistercian cloister in Syrian Tripoli.[36] Nonetheless, it took Europe by storm in the last years of the thirteenth century, no doubt because it so accurately "foretold" the fall of Tripoli and Acre (in fact, more prophecy after the event) and placed those events within a larger prophetic context. Around the time of the Black Death it could be found in numerous libraries and obviously appeared to someone to contain accurate predictions of current events — namely, the coming of "plagues in many places," and the coming of a "people without a head," who could be seen as the flagellants ("without a head" because they had no known leader).[37] Since the vision "predicted" the present so well, the unknown reader must have decided that here was a certain guide to the future and therefore decided to circulate it for the benefit of his contemporaries. Instead of recirculating it untouched, however, he rewrote the introduction to state that the Cistercian monk saw his vision in Tripoli in 1347.[38] Surely he did this to make his vision seem more immediate, but he clearly did not give his alteration much careful thought: in 1347 the Holy Land had been lost for more than a half-century, and it was ridiculous to imagine a Cistercian cloister there or a message predicting the fall of cities that had long since fallen.

Still, the version of the "Cedar of Lebanon" prophecy for 1347, which otherwise contained only minor revisions, was an enormous success. There are at least ten surviving manuscript copies, and the textual variants that appear in these copies are so multifarious that there could easily have been more than one hundred copies now lost.[39] (Short prophecies sometimes circulated on single sheets that were not subsequently preserved.) The ten copies also bear witness to a very wide geographical distribution, having been copied in places as distant from each other as Ireland, England, Catalonia, the Rhineland, and Lower Austria.[40] Some of the copies were made after the plague subsided, but some circulated while the epidemic was raging: the copy from Lilienfeld, Lower Austria, concludes with a report of the desolation wrought by the plague in Avignon. Like John of Bassigny's prophecy and the rumors reported by William of Blofield, the revised version of the "Cedar of Lebanon" vision must have been conceived in order to relate the woes of the present to the certainties of the future. Despite its chronological absurdities, it circulated widely because it helped many to fathom the otherwise unfathomable.[41]

The wide circulation of the "Cedar of Lebanon" vision makes it abundantly clear that the chiliastic prophecies were not exclusively spread by flagellants, or (if at all) by "fanatics" or heretics who tried to play on the despondency of the dislocated lower classes. None of the copies was accompanied by any call for violent action, and all whose provenance can be determined came from monastic or aristocratic milieux. Similarly, John of Bassigny's prophecy was transmitted and studied by clerics,[42] and William of Blofield said nothing about the rumors he reported having been spread by flagellants, rabble-rousers, or heretics. If we include the prophecy of Michael de Leone's "great astrologer" in the list of chiliastic texts inspired by the plague, we have still another prophecy that traveled in thoroughly respectable and orthodox circles.

All of this should not be surprising since it was obviously not necessary to be aberrant and poor to be upset by the plague, and resort to prophecy was meant to provide edification and comfort, not inspiration for insurrection. Europeans tried to comprehend the fury of the plague with the aid of what might be called a prophetic "deep structure." The prophecies I have introduced were certainly conceived independently, but, aside from variations in details, all foresaw contemporary storms being succeeded by wondrous times of peace and Christian triumph. One might make an analogy to the calm after the storm in Beethoven's *Pastoral* Symphony, were it not for the fact that the prophetic calm after the storm was not the finale but was expected to be followed by either the reign of Antichrist or the advent of Gog and Magog, with the Last Judgment to follow in either case thereafter. Peace and tranquillity on earth might be great but earthly attainments could never be perfect or eternal, for Christianity was based on the assumption that perfection could only be found in the hereafter and the beyond.

The reasons for the similarities in the plague prophecies were probably twofold. First, as we have seen, fully developed prophetic traditions lay behind all of the texts. Despite his assertion of sudden illumination, Rupescissa's predictions rested on a long tradition of post-Antichrist eschatological exegesis, and prophecies of coming messianic rulers and times of peace before Antichrist had circulated in Christian Europe before 1347. Within certain limits prophets were free to alter details: they might state that the coming new age would be longer or shorter or that it would have more of one kind of progressive fulfillment than another. But within both the post- and pre-Antichrist alternatives there were basic sequences of events that prophets were virtually obliged to follow.

And, second, just those basic sequences were designed to provide comfort. Present disasters might be tolerated better if they could be viewed in terms of a coherent divine plan. Chastisements might come, but it was surely comforting to know that they would have an end and be followed by "peace and tranquillity." So whenever new disasters struck — the Black Death is by no means the only example[43] — new prophecies were brought forth out of the "deep structure" or old prophecies were retailored to fit new events.

Mentalities, Like Mediterranean sailing routes, have their *longues durées*. The Black Death, medieval Europe's greatest disaster, prompted many to think about how the present related to the future and called forth expressions of chiliasm that circulated from Italy to England and from Austria to Catalonia. In their main outlines, these expressions were not new but were manifestations of a basically unchanging medieval prophetic structure. They were meant to inspire perseverance in faith, hope, and penance, but they were not otherwise meant as calls to action. They intended to give comfort by providing certainties in the face of uncertainty and must have helped frightened Europeans get about their work.[44] In such ways can mentalities, like sailing routes, support life.

Appendix

William of Blofield's Report of Rumors from Roman Parts

I edit the following from Cambridge, Corpus Christi College, MS 404, f. 102r-v. For a description of the manuscript, see M. R. James, *A Descriptive Catalogue of the Manuscripts in the Library of Corpus Christi College, Cambridge*, 2 (Cambridge, 1912): 269-77; and, for further information on the manuscript, see Rouse, "Bostonus Buriensis and the Author of the *Catalogus Scriptorum Ecclesiae*," 475, *passim*; and Reeves, *Influence of Prophecy in the Later Middle Ages*, 539. Reeves edited the first half of the text; ibid, 94. I adhere to the spelling of the manuscript, except in providing "v" for consonantal "u," but I have modernized the punctuation and capitalization.

> Subscriptos rumores scripsit frater Willelmus de Blofeld in Anglia, anno Domini m.ccc.xlix, cuidam fratri conventus Fratrum Predicatorum Norwicensis, quod prophete diversi sunt in partibus Romanorum, sed adhuc occulti, qui omnia fictiva predixerunt per annos multos. Et isto anno, videlicet ab incarnacione m.ccc.xlix, predicant Antichristum habere se x annos etatis et puerum esse dilectissimum et doctissimum in omni sciencia, in tantum quod non est aliquis iam vivens qui sibi poterit coequari. Predicant eciam alium puerum ultra Tartaros iam natum xii annorum, qui in fide Christiana est imbutus, et hic est qui perfidiam Saracenorum destruet et maximus est inter Christianos, sed cito finietur eius imperium in adventu Antichristi. Isti eciam prophete de isto papa inter cetera dicunt quod finem violencium faciet. Dicunt eciam quod post mortem istius pape tot revoluciones erunt in mundo quot nunquam fuerunt per aliquod tempus. Sed post hec surget alius papa bonus et iustus, et cardinales creabit dominum timentes, et tempore huius maxime erit pax. Et post eum nullus erit papa, sed Antichristus veniet et se ostendet, etc.

notes

This paper, originally delivered at the Binghamton Black Death conference, was first published in the *American Historical Review*, 86 (1981): 533–52 and is here reprinted with some minor changes. The author has benefited from criticism by Charles M. Radding and Michael Barkun, from review of transcriptions by Daniel Williman, and from editorial improvements offered by Anne Lee Bain. Research expenses were generously funded by the National Endowment for the Humanities, the American Council of Learned Societies, and Northwestern University. Abbreviations used in the footnotes include the following: BL — British Library, London; BN — Bibliothèque Nationale, Paris; *MGH — Monumenta Germaniae Historica*; and Töpfer, *Reich des Friedens* — Bernhard Töpfer, *Das kommende Reich des Friedens* (Berlin, 1964).

1. Foster, "Assessing Disaster Magnitude," *Professional Geographer*, 28 (1976): 241–47.

2. Mathias von Neuenburg, *Chronica*, ed. A. Hofmeister, in *MGH, Scriptores rerum Germanicarum*, new ser., 4:263–64; and *La Vita di Cola di Rienzo*, ed. A. M. Ghisalberti (Rome, 1928): bk. 2, chap. 3, as translated in John Wright, *The Life of Cola di Rienzo* (Toronto, 1975), 103.

3. As-Sulūk, as quoted in Michael W. Dols, *The Black Death in the Middle East* (Princeton, 1977), 290.

4. *Detmar–Chronik*, in C. Hegel, ed., *Die Chroniken der deutschen Städte vom 14. bis ins 16. Jahrhundert* (Leipzig, etc., 1862-), 19:522: ". . . so sint desse stervende, orloghe, vorretnisse unde al de plaghe, de nù scheen, mer de tekene, de Cristus heft ghesproken in den hilgen ewangelien, dat se scholen scheen vor der lesten tiid; wo langhe vore, dat is nicht beschreven, wente Gode is dat alleneghen bekant"; and Johannes Vitoduranus, *Chronica*, ed. F. Baethgen, in *MGH, Scriptores rerum Germanicarum*, new ser., 3:276: "Predicta, scilicet terre motus et pestilencia, precurrencia mala sunt extreme voraginis et tempestatis secundum verbum salvatoris in ewangelio dicentis: 'Erunt terre motus per loca et pestilencia et fames' et cetera." Also see n. 35 below, an attack of 1348 against speculations about the birth of Antichrist in the unpublished *Monastica* of Conrad of Megenberg, as quoted in Sabine Krüger, "Krise der Zeit als Ursache der Pest?" in *Festschrift für Hermann Heimpel*, 2 (Göttingen, 1972): 857.

5. Haupt, "Kirchliche Geisselung und Geisslerbruderschaften," in *Realencyklopädie für protestantische Theologie und Kirche*, 6 (Leipzig, 1899): 437; Cohn, *The Pursuit of the Millennium* (1957; 3d ed., New York, 1970), 136–39; Ziegler, *The Black Death* (1969; reprint ed., New York, 1971), 92; and Erbstösser, *Sozialreligiöse Strömungen im späten Mittelalter* (Berlin, 1970), 32. Karl Müller had already criticized a first attempt by Haupt to demonstrate flagellant millenarianism; Müller, "Die Arbeiten zur Kirchengeschichte des 14. und 15. Jahrhunderts," *Zeitschrift für Kirchengeschichte*, 7 (1885): 113–14.

6. Kieckhefer, "Radical Tendencies in the Flagellant Movement of the Mid-Fourteenth Century," *Journal of Medieval and Renaissance Studies*, 4 (1974): 157–76, at 167–69. Kieckhefer has convincingly argued for the exclusion of other texts that have previously been adduced to demonstrate the alleged millenarianism of the flagellants. Siegfried Hoyer's claim that the flagellants of 1349 "followed the directives of a prophet" rests on a mistranslation of a fifteenth-century Dutch text, as in Paul Fredericq, *Corpus documentorum inquisitionis haereticae pravitatis Neerlandicae*, 1 (Ghent, 1899): 197; see Hoyer, "Die thüringsche Kryptoflagellantenbewegung im 15. Jahrhundert," *Jahrbuch für Regionalgeschichte*, 2 (1967): 148–74, at 161.

7. The *questio* from the Breslau manuscript remains unedited, but Erbstösser has published the part concerning the flagellants; *Sozialreligiöse Strömungen im späten Mittelalter*, 27–28 n. 82. The relevant section reads "Item de quadam sua cantilena dicebant quod post 17 annos immediate

presentem annum domini 1349 sequentes religiones et precipue mendicantium ordines post multas [Erbstösser: "multis"] tribulationes deficient substituto quodam novo ordine. Postquam etiam priores ordines cum magna gloria resuscitabuntur et tunc mundus certissime finietur. . . ."

8. Kieckhefer, "Radical Tendencies in the Flagellant Movement," 167–69. Erbstösser speculated that remarks about the Hussites might have been added later but gave no grounds for concluding that they were; *Sozialreligiöse Strömungen im späten Mittelalter*, 27.

9. Cohn, *The Pursuit of the Millennium*, 137. Erbstösser has called attention to another of Cohn's mistakes—namely, the assumption that, since the *questio* is found in a manuscript now in Breslau, it must have pertained to flagellants who were there; in fact, the manuscript was almost certainly copied in Erfurt; *Sozialreligiöse Strömungen im späten Mittelalter*, 26.

10. Fritsche Closener, *Strassburgische Chronik*, in Hegel, *Die Chroniken der deutschen Städte*, 8: 114: "So wil ich uber üch dún minen heiligen segen, so bringet daz ertrich früht mit gnoden und würt alle die welt erfullet mit miner wirdekeit." Kieckhefer has found a lack of millenarianism in the heavenly letter, but he did not deal explicitly with this passage; "Radical Tendencies in the Flagellant Movement," 168.

11. Erbstösser, *Sozialreligiöse Strömungen im späten Mittelalter*, 46, n. 157, citing the research of R. Priebsch. Bernhard Töpfer stated succinctly that the apparently chiliastic passage in this heavenly letter represents "recht unbestimmter Hoffnungen . . . ein ausgeprägt joachimitisches Gepräge zeigen diese Erwartungen allerdings nicht"; Töpfer, *Reich des Friedens*, 282–83.

12. Gordon Leff, *Heresy in the Later Middle Ages: The Relation of Heterodoxy to Dissent, c. 1250–c. 1450*, 2 (New York, 1967): 488–89.

13. On the definition of chiliasm (or millenarianism) I follow, among many others, Norman Cohn, "Medieval Millenarism," in Sylvia L. Thrupp, ed., *Millennial Dreams in Action* (New York, 1970), 31; Y. Talmon, "Millenarian Movements,"*European Journal of Sociology*, 7 (1966): 200, as cited in Clarke Garrett, *Respectable Folly: Millenarians and the French Revolution in France and England* (Baltimore, 1975), 1; and Michael Barkun, *Disaster and the Millennium* (New Haven, 1974), 18. Earlier scholarship, particularly under Cohn's influence, was primarily interested in finding a chiliasm that expresses "an active desire to speed the inevitable result, often through violent, revolutionary means"; Barkun, *Disaster and the Millennium*, 18. In the last few years, however, some scholars have been paying more attention to chiliasm's passive or conservative face. Bryan W. Ball, for example, has emphasized that "a millenarian was not, *ipso facto*, a heretic or even necessarily an extremist"; Ball, *A Great Expectation: Eschatological Thought in English Protestantism to 1660* (Leiden, 1975), 233. For an excellent bibliographical review that points to a trend away from the preoccupation with revolutionary chiliasm and assumptions of psychopathology, see Hillel Schwartz, "The End of the Beginning: Millenarian Studies, 1969–1975," *Religious Studies Review*, 2, no. 3 (1976): 1–15 (kindly called

to my attention by Professor Kieckhefer). Bernard McGinn, in an anthology that appeared after this paper was written, has preferred the word apocalypticism to millenarianism or chiliasm but agreed that "beliefs about the coming age . . . were as important for social continuity as they were for social change . . . , as often designed to maintain the political, social, and economic order as to overthrow it"; McGinn, *Visions of the End: Apocalyptic Traditions in the Middle Ages* (New York, 1979), 28–36, at 30.

14. The terminology is my own. I developed the distinction, expanding on the work of Marjorie Reeves's *The Influence of Prophecy in the Later Middle Ages* (Oxford, 1969), in my "Refreshment of the Saints: The Time after Antichrist as a Station for Earthly Progress in Medieval Thought," *Traditio*, 32 (1976): 97–144. Documented support for what I say in this and the following two paragraphs appears in that article. "Post-" and "pre-Antichrist" should not be confused with "post-" and "premillennial," terms that refer to debates among early modern and modern millenarian theologians about whether the second advent of Christ would come after or before the millennium. Medieval "pre-Antichrist" chiliasm did not address itself to the pre- or postmillennial question at all, and medieval "post-Antichrist" theologians differed as to whether the millennium to come after Antichrist would be brought in directly by Christ's second advent or not.

15. For the only reliable original survey of Rupescissa's life and prophetic thought, see Jeanne Bignami-Odier, *Etudes sur Jean de Roquetaillade (Johannes de Rupescissa)* (Paris, 1952); and, for the *Liber secretorum eventuum* specifically, see ibid., 113–29. Marjorie Reeves has provided an English summary of Bignami-Odier's work; *Influence of Prophecy in the Later Middle Ages*, 225–28, 321–24. Lynn Thorndike has edited the chapter headings of the *Liber secretorum eventuum* as they appear in BN, MS lat. 3598; see Thorndike, *A History of Magic and Experimental Science*, 3 (New York, 1934): 722–25. For a description of this manuscript, see Bignami-Odier, *Etudes sur Jean de Roquetaillade*, 239–40.

16. BN, MS lat. 3598, f. 4r-v: "Quarto intellexi multas clades futuras erunt in ianuis et evenire validas tempestates. Primo famem generalem simul cum mortalitate in orbe que facta est anno Domini M°ccc°xlvii° per seculum universum. Secundo multiplicacionem innumerabilium cadaverorum anno Christi M°ccc°xlviii° ubique terrarum multifarie [MS: "multifamine"] dispersorum."

17. For Rupescissa's arrest, imprisonment in Figeac, and revelation of July 1345, see Bignami-Odier, *Etudes sur Jean de Roquetaillade*, 17–18 (drawing upon Rupescissa's *Liber Ostensor* of 1356), 114 (translating from Rupescissa's *Liber secretorum eventuum*). To my knowledge, Rupescissa was the first medieval writer to espouse literal chiliasm or millennialism; I intend to write further on this and other noteworthy themes in Rupescissa's prophecies.

18. Bignami-Odier, *Etudes sur Jean de Roquetaillade*, 20.

19. Rupescissa, Commentary on the *Oraculum Cyrilli*, written over several years between 1345 and 1349, BN, MS lat. 2599, f. 167v: "Nota quod

a. D. Mcccxlviii, qui est annus pestis magne ire Dei, vidi coram me quod-dam genus muscarum. . . ."

20. In addition to the three Latin copies and Catalan translation listed by Bignami-Odier (238–42), there are also two hitherto unnoticed Latin copies: Turin, Biblioteca Nazionale Universitaria, MS K² IV 13, ff. 137r–67v (mid-fifteenth century); and Milan, Biblioteca Trivulziana, MS n. 199, ff. 21v–29r (year 1496). The German chronicler Conrad of Halberstadt presented a resumé of the *Liber secretorum eventuum* which he saw in Avignon in 1353. The *Liber secretorum eventuum* was also known to the author of the *Chronographia regum Francorum* and to Jean le Bel. Bignami-Odier, *Etudes sur Jean de Roquetaillade*, 113, 127 n. 3, 219, 221, 233–34. A complete manuscript abbreviation is in Rouen MS 1355, ff. 90r–91r (ca. 1400); and, for extracts, in addition to those in the manuscripts listed by Bignami-Odier, see Basel MS F V 6, f. 130v (ca. 1420) and Tours MS 520, ff. 47v–48r (year 1422). A fifteenth-century marginaliast in the Tours manuscript refers to having another complete parchment copy. (I used a microfilm of Tours MS 520 generously lent to me by the Institut de Recherche et d'Histoire des Textes, Paris.)

21. For an excellent survey of such prophecies that circulated before the fourteenth century, see Töpfer, *Reich des Friedens*, esp. chaps. 1, 4.

22. Erbstösser's finding of chiliastic expectations in verses added to the *Chronica S. Petri Erfordensis* is untenable: these do not refer to a "returned Frederick" but merely to the succession of Margrave Friedrich III of Meissen on the death of his father, Margrave Friedrich II; for Erbstösser's remark, see *Sozialreligiöse Strömungen im späten Mittelalter*, 32.

23. Vitoduranus, *Chronica*, 280–81. For an English translation, see McGinn, *Visions of the End*, 251; for the best of the numerous treatments of this passage, see Töpfer, *Reich des Friedens*, 178–82. John's chronicle stops in 1348, before the Black Death had spread to Germany.

24. Michael de Leone, *Annotata historica* [more properly, *De cronicis temporum modernorum hominum*], ed. J. F. Böhmer, *Fontes rerum Germanicarum*, 1 (1843; reprint ed., Aalen, 1969): 474. For the dating of Michael's history to June 1349, see Stuart Jenks, "The Black Death and Würzburg: Michael de Leone's Reaction in Context" (Ph.D. dissertation, Yale University, 1976), 37.

25. Stuart Jenks has observantly noticed that the "great astrologer's" prediction "unus solus erit dominus" echoes Ezekiel 37:22 — "rex unus erit dominus" — which, according to Vitoduranus, *Chronica*, 281, was a prediction cited to express hopes for the return of Frederick II around 1348; Jenks, "Die Prophezeiung von Ps.-Hildegard von Bingen: Eine vernachlässigte Quelle über die Geisslerzüge von 1348/49," *Mainfränkisches Jahrbuch*, 29 (1977): 9–38, at 35 n. 51.

26. The only prior published treatments, excluding the fanciful nineteenth-century ones (see note 33, pp. 101 f., below), are Noël Valois, "Conseils et prédictions adressés à Charles VII, en 1445, par un certain Jean du Bois," *Annuaire-Bulletin de la Société de l'Histoire de France*, 46 (1909):

201–38, at 223–25; and Thorndike, *A History of Magic and Experimental Science*, 312–15. Valois referred to John only insofar as he is used by the fifteenth-century Jean du Bois; Thorndike treated John's prophecy more extensively but without knowledge of the prophetic tradition within which John worked and without sufficient knowledge of the extant manuscripts. Valois and Thorndike knew two copies of John of Bassigny's prophecy: BN, MS lat. 7352, ff. 2r–4v (fifteenth century); and Tours MS 520, ff. 146r–49v (year 1422). I have relied on Valois's and Thorndike's works for readings from the Bibliothèque Nationale manuscript. I have found four more copies that are independent of the late *Mirabilis Liber* printed version (note 33, p. 101 f., below): Kues, Hospitalbibliothek, MS 57, ff. 103vb–4rb (first half of the fifteenth century) (Sara Clark kindly lent me a microfilm of this copy); Bamberg, Staatsbibliothek, MS Msc. Astr. 4, ff. 155r–57v (first half of the fifteenth century) (f. 157 is bound out of order; it should precede f. 155); BL, MS Cotton, Cleopatra C IV, ff. 81v–85v (late fifteenth century); and BL, MS Lansdowne 762, ff. 54v–57v (early sixteenth century). The last two copies are too corrupt to be of help in establishing readings, but the Kues and Bamberg texts are important witnesses. Unfortunately, the Kues copy breaks off less than halfway through the text; I follow it where I can and use the Bamberg copy for the rest. Another valuable independent witness is provided by hitherto unnoticed reports from the Bassigny prophecy in the mid-fifteenth century chronicle of Adrien de But, Cistercian of Dunes (West Flanders): see his *Chronique*, ed. Kervyn de Lettenhove, *Chroniques relatives à l'histoire de la Belgique sous la domination des ducs de Bourgogne: 1, Chroniques des religieux des Dunes* (Brussels, 1870), pp. 284, 296, 302–4, 529. A complete study and critical edition of the prophecy would be a valuable contribution to prophetic and mid-fourteenth-century French history.

27. In the Bibliothèque Nationale manuscript, John claimed to have spoken with a Syrian in "Gadis subtus Quadrum," with a Chaldean in "Bethsedin iuxta Montem Thabor," and with a Jew in "garda Ademari"; BN, MS lat. 7352, as given by Valois, "Conseils et prédictions adressés à Charles VII," 223 n. 1. So far as I can see, the Kues, Bamberg, and Tours manuscripts all omit reference to the Jew and give, respectively, the following forms for the first two place names: "Gradris subtus Quadum," "Betseladim iuxta Montem Tabor"; "Gadzis subtus Quadrum," "Bethseladum iuxta Montem Thabor"; and "Gadris subtus Cadrum," "Seboch iuxta Montem Thabor." Of all these names, the only one that appears in Graesse-Benedict's *Orbis Latinus* is Bethsedin — the biblical Bethsaida — which is near, but not immediately next to, Mount Tabor. N. B.: After this went to press I realized that *Gardu Ademari* is surely Garde-Adhémar in Dauphine (Drôme; arrond. Montélimar), that *Gradis* must be Gaza, and that *Quadrum* is very likely Darum; apparently, then, John's place names were not bogus after all!

28. Compare Valois, "Conseils et prédictions adressés à Charles VII," 223 n. 1: ". . . prédictions rédigées entre les années 1342 et 1345." Thorn-

dike, *A History of Magic and Experimental Science*, 3: 314, is properly more skeptical.

29. Kues, Hospitalbibliothek, MS 57, f. 104ra: "Nam idem ille annus Domini Mcccxliii erit inicium omnium dolorum, quoniam in ipso anno incipiet et eveniet quedam generalis mortalitas et pestis que universum mundum mutabiliter vexabit et affliget, ita quod bene fere plusquam media pars, velut verius dicere due partes, hominum mundi morientur. Et infra quadragesimum quintum mensem, que pestis pro certo xlv menses durabit, vel amplius, licet regnet et vadat modo ibi, modo alibi." Although the Kues manuscript has "Mcccxliii," 1344 is meant because the prior sentence refers to troubles beginning "ab anno Mcccxliii in anno proximo"; the reading of 1344 is confirmed by the Bamberg manuscript, a marginal note in the Tours manuscript, and Adrien de But, 284.

30. The term "Black Death" was not a contemporary one; chroniclers usually used the terms "grandis mortalitas" or "grandis pestis"; see Dols, *The Black Death in the Middle East*, 5 n. 5.

31. The Bibliothèque Nationale copy that Thorndike used has 1382, but I follow the Bamberg manuscript, which consistently presents the most coherent dates.

32. Bamberg, Staatsbibliothek, MS Msc. Astr. 4, f. 156r: "Ordinabit autem Deus secum unum imperatorem sanctissimum qui erit de reliquiis et nobilissimi sanguinis et seminis Francorum regum. Et erit sibi in adiutorium et obediens in omnibus mandatis eius ad reformandum in melius universum orbem. Sub ipsis autem papa et imperatore pacificabitur omnis orbis, quoniam ira Domini quiescet; et sic erit una lex, una vita, et una fides, et erunt homines unanimes, et invicem se amantes, et concordantes. Durabitque pax per annos multos. Postquam autem seculo in melius reformato, iterum multa signa in celo apparebunt qua malicia hominum se evigilabit, et ad mala pristina et malicias pessimas homines revertentur . . . et tunc apparebit Antichristus."

33. P. Meyvaert, "John Erghome and the *Vaticinium Roberti Bridlington*," *Speculum*, 41 (1966): 656–64, at 658; and Reeves, *Influence of Prophecy in the Later Middle Ages*, 254–56. A bizarre resurrection of the Bassigny prophecy in revolutionary and postrevolutionary France is worth a full study but may be alluded to briefly here. The story begins with the publication of a very corrupt version of the text, ascribed to "Johannes de Vatiguerro," in the *Mirabilis Liber*, a patriotic French prophetic anthology published at least six times in Paris in the 1520s and once in Rome in 1524. (Occasional reference to a Venetian edition of 1514 is clearly a bibliographical error. Dated Parisian editions appeared in 1522, 1523, and 1524, and at least three others were published around the same time in Paris without date "au Pellican," "au Roi David," and "à l'Eléphant." In the undated "au Pellican" edition, the "Vatiguerrus" prophecy appears at folios 55r–58r; in the Rome edition it is at folios 46r–48v.) Centuries later, in 1795, a French Royalist who read the "Vatiguerrus" prophecy in a copy of the *Mirabilis Liber* he found in Paris in the Bibliothèque Nationale concluded

that it applied perfectly to the present tribulations of France and also foretold a Bourbon restoration. The results were that many others flooded the Bibliothèque Nationale to read the notorious prediction, that the police cracked down and imprisoned a librarian for making the *Mirabilis Liber* available, and that copies of the "Vatiguerrus" prophecy circulated clandestinely throughout France in a tendentiously altered version fathered on St. Cesarius of Arles. After the Restoration the prophecy could once more go public, and thus in 1814 and 1815, and then again after the Revolutions of 1830 and 1848, numerous editions appeared of either the "Cesarius" text or the unaltered "Vatiguerrus" one, printed in Latin or French or in both languages simultaneously. For an illustrative example, see [Hyacinthe Olivier-Vitalis, ed.] *Prophétie recuellie et transmise par Jean de Vatiguerro; extraite du Liber Mirabilis* (Carpentras 1814); I have used a copy in Avignon, Bibliothèque Calvet, In–8°24,897. Olivier-Vitalis explained how, as librarian at Carpentras, he had earlier hidden away three copies of the *Mirabilis Liber* to make sure that the police would not confiscate them and how he was now free to bring out the "Vatiguerrus" text publicly in Latin with facing-page French, together with a commentary showing how it accurately predicted, among other things, the death of Louis XVI, the persecution of the Church, and the return of the Bourbons, to be followed by a long reign of peace. For more, but by no means exhaustive, information on the "Vatiguerrus"-"Cesarius" copies, see Abbé Lecanu, *Dictionnaire des prophéties et des miracles,* 2 (Paris, 1852): 54–61, 716; and Jean Harmand, "Une Prophétie du XVIᵉ siècle sur la Révolution," *Revue des études historiques,* 79 (1913): 523–49. Neither Lecanu nor Harmand knew that the "Vatiguerrus" prophecy was originally written in the fourteenth century by John of Bassigny.

34. Cambridge, Corpus Christi College, MS 404, f.102; I edit this text in the appendix, pp. 94–95. Marjorie Reeves edited without comment the first half of this text; *Influence of Prophecy in the Later Middle Ages,* 94. On William, see A. B. Emden, *A Biographical Register of the University of Cambridge to 1500* (Cambridge, 1963), 66. Emden has shown that William belonged to the Carmelite convent of Cambridge in 1343. Although the Cambridge text presents some ambiguity, I prefer to think that William sent his report to Norwich from Italy rather than from some place in England. (It is noteworthy that Blofield is only about ten kilometers away from Norwich; the recipient of William's report may have been a relative or local friend.) On the copyist of the Cambridge manuscript, Henry of Kirkestede, who was the librarian of Bury St. Edmunds, see Richard H. Rouse, "Bostonus Buriensis and the Author of the *Catalogus Scriptorum Ecclesiae,*" *Speculum,* 41 (1966): 471–99. Henry found William of Blofield's report in Norwich on his bibliographical travels and expressed his own doubts about the rumors by writing in the margin of his copy *mendacium.* My study of the manuscript in connection with the "Cedar of Lebanon" prophecy leads me to believe that Henry's copy dates from between ca. 1365 and ca. 1377; for the "Cedar of Lebanon" prophecy, see note 35, page 103, below.

35. For published editions of versions close to the one used by the mid-fourteenth-century reviser, see *MGH, Scriptores rerum Germanicarum*, 17:605, and 23:567–68. My forthcoming *Powers of Prophecy: The Cedar of Lebanon Vision from the Mongol Onslaught to the Dawn of the Enlightenment* will provide editions and more information concerning the various versions. Independent evidence that people during the time of the plague resorted to old prophecies to make sense of current events comes from the plague entry for 1348 in the German vernacular *Oberrheinischen Chronik*, ed. H. Maschek, *Deutsche Chroniken* (Leipzig, 1936), 64, as quoted by Martin Haeusler, *Das Ende der Geschichte in der mittelalterlichen Weltchronistik* (Cologne, 1980), 121: "Und meinet men, das die prophecien Apocalipsis und Hiltgardis [Hildegard of Bingen] und ander prophecien von dem iungesten tage und von dem endecrist nie so gar wurdent erfüllet als dis iores."

36. See my "Medieval Prophecy and Religious Dissent," *Past & Present*, no. 72 (1976): 3–24, at 12.

37. For an explicit statement that the "people without a head" in the prophecy were the flagellants, see Breslau (Wrocław), University Library, MS IV F 6, f. 100v; for a published edition, see Joseph Klapper, ed., *Exempla aus Handschriften des Mittelalters* (Heidelberg, 1911), 64 (which was kindly called to my attention by Dr. P. Dinzelbacher, Stuttgart). For independent designations of the flagellants as "gens sine capite," also see Erbstösser, *Sozialreligiöse Strömungen im späten Mittelalter*, 27; and Jenks, "Die Prophezeiung von Ps.-Hildegard von Bingen," 20.

38. For the only published edition of this version, see Jean Leclercq, "Textes et manuscrits cisterciens dans des bibliothèques des Etats-Unis," *Traditio*, 17 (1961): 163–83, at 166–69. The manuscript that Leclercq used gives the date 1346 for the vision, but I believe this to be a variant from the original revision's 1347. Leclercq's commentary is based on the fallacious assumption that the single copy he used was unique.

39. The ten medieval copies I know are *The Annals of Ireland by Friar John Clyn*, ed. Richard Butler (Dublin, 1849), 36 (information courtesy of Mr. John R. Shinners, University of Toronto); Oxford, Bodleian Library, MS Bodley 761, f. 184v (Frau Waltraud Huber kindly called my attention to this copy); Oxford, Bodleian Library, MS Digby 218, f. 107r; Oxford, Bodleian Library, MS. Fairfax 27, f. 26r; Oxford, Bodleian Library, MS Hatton 56, f. 32v; BN, MS Français 902, f. 96v; Yale University Library, MS Marston 225, ff. 43v–44v (the copy that Leclercq edited); Munich, Bayerische Staatsbibliothek, MS Clm 28229, f. 21r; Lilienfeld MS 49, f. 357r (a copy I learned of by means of the incipit list of the Hill Monastic Manuscript Library, St. John's University, Collegeville, Minn.); and Carpentras MS 336, ff. 75v–76v (a Catalan translation). A seventeenth-century copy of the Fairfax 27 text appears in Oxford, Bodleian Library, MS Fairfax 28, f. iii^v.

40. The Clyn copy is from Kilkenny, Ireland and the Bodleian ones all from England; the Carpentras copy is from Catalonia; the Munich copy is from Speyer on the Rhine (I am grateful to Dr. Alexander Patch-

ovsky for this identification); and the Lilienfeld copy is from Lilienfeld, Lower Austria.

41. Another prophecy that may have been redated to relate to the Black Death derives from the *De semine scripturarum*. In the original version of this early thirteenth-century work, which is still unedited, the time of the letter "x" (in which the Church was to be cleansed of corruption) was to last from 1215 to 1315, and the time of the letter "y" (one of the conversion of all peoples) from 1315 to 1415. See Töpfer, *Reich des Friedens*, 46; and H. Grundmann, "Ueber die Schriften des Alexander von Roes," *Deutsches Archiv für Erforschung des Mittelalters*, 8 (1950): 162. But in a Würzburg University Library manuscript (Mp. mi. f. 6, f. 37r), the time of "x" is altered to the years 1248 to 1348, and of "y" to the years 1348 to 1448; see H. Grauert, *Magister Heinrich der Poet in Würzburg und die römische Kurie*, Abhandlungen der königlichen Bayerischen Akademie der Wissenschaften, philos.-philol. und hist. Klasse, 27, 1–2 (Munich, 1912), 443–44. Also see Jenks, "Die Prophezeiung von Ps.-Hildegard von Bingen," 17, 35 n. 54. Jenks has read the date given for the prophecy of Merlin in the manuscript following the references to *De semine scripturarum* as 1343; but to my mind this dating does not necessarily conflict with Grauert's view that the text was copied around 1350. Since the manuscript was written under the direction of Michael de Leone, it is possible that the redating was done by Michael or someone shortly before him as a way of reconceiving the prophecy in terms of a newly perceived significance found in the plague. Further study of the textual traditions of *De semine scripturarum* might help confirm or disprove this hypothesis.

42. Both the Augustinian friar John Erghome and the parish priest Guillaume Bauge of Nouans in the diocese of Tours, whose copy was used for the edition in the *Mirabilis Liber*, studied John of Bassigny's prophecy. The copy of Bassigny's prophecy in the Tours manuscript collection was made in the Benedictine monastery of Marmoutier. On John Erghome, see Meyvaert, "John Erghome and the *Vaticinium Roberti Bridlington*," 656–64; and Reeves, *Influence of Prophecy in the Later Middle Ages*, 254–56.

43. For three prophecies in addition to the "Cedar of Lebanon" text that seem to have been inspired by the fall of Tripoli and Acre, see my "Medieval Prophecy and Religious Dissent," 14. Numerous examples of other prophecies inspired by other disasters or portents could be adduced. The Black Death itself seems to have inspired fewer prophecies than one might have expected, but as yet this is only an impression; perhaps other prophecies circulated that are still unidentified or lost, and perhaps some older prophecies were applied by contemporaries to the Black Death in ways that are still unknown. A comparison between the number and nature of prophecies inspired by the Black Death and other events that were perceived to be disastrous might be instructive; but at present that project seems too difficult to undertake.

44. Compare M. Dols, "Comparative Communal Responses to the Black Death in Muslim and Christian Societies," *Viator*, 5 (1974): 269–87; and

his *Black Death in the Middle East*, 281–302. Dols has emphasized the contemporary Islamic lack of eschatological hopes and consequent resignation and fatalism. Despite Dols's thoughtful work, comparisons between Western Christian and Islamic reactions to the plague must remain highly speculative, owing to the deficiencies of the sources and the complexities of the problem.

Aspects of the Fourteenth-Century Iconography of Death and the Plague

Joseph Polzer

After an absence of about 600 years the plague struck Europe with devastating force in 1348, and returned periodically thereafter until modern times. It is estimated that the Black Death of 1348 killed about one-fourth to one-third of the population of western Europe. The effect of its drastic reappearance on the stage of Europe, and how this catastrophe challenged the social fabric and the human spirit, is the theme of this symposium.

We focus on the late medieval fascination with natural death and decay. The Christian idea, we underscore, sees the dead rising in the flesh at the Last Judgment, spiritually alive to receive a reward or punishment earned in life: an eternity in heaven or hell. This moral drama, requiring psychologically aware and physiologically animate actors, is antithetical to the obliteraton of life which is evident in the cycle of nature in its normal course, and which is underscored by mortal epidemic disease.

The view largely prevails that the extreme and indiscriminate mortality of the Black Death influenced the late medieval preoccupation with natural death. This is unquestionable. However, in the light of the Christian alternative, which considers death the gateway to eternal life, the extent and character of this nexus remain to be more closely studied, as it bears on reason and the search for rational cause and control, on faith and the fatalistic acceptance of God's wrath, and on the fascination with natural death and decay which, as we shall see, was gathering momentum before the Black Death struck.

The most impressive contemporary representation of Death's power is the fresco known as the *Triumph of Death* in the Campo

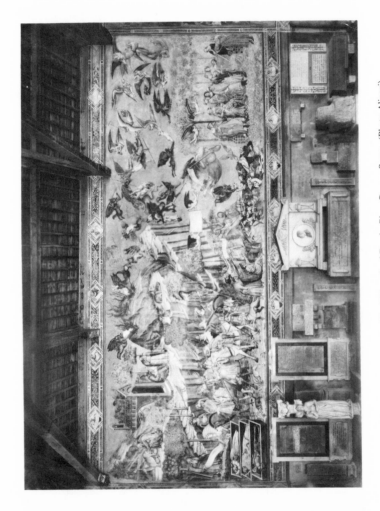

Fig. 1. Francesco Traini, The Triumph of Death. Pisa, Campo Santo. (Photo Alinari)

Santo in Pisa (fig. 1). Until recently, its drastic prose was considered by virtually all scholars to reflect the plague of 1348, and this view still largely prevails. It is shared by Millard Meiss in his important book on the art of Tuscany during the later Trecento,[1] by Frederick Hartt in his recent textbook on Italian Renaissance art,[2] by Hellmut Rosenfeld in a recent edition of his *Mittelalterliche Totentanz*,[3] and by Robert Oertel in his fine *Early Italian Painting to 1400*,[4] just to mention a few examples which guide general scholarly opinion. The mid-nineteen-sixties, however, witnessed a change in perspective. Since then the Pisan *Triumph of Death* (and the fresco cycle to which it belongs) has been placed by a number of specialists before the great pandemic.[5] Clearly, this has a fundamental bearing on our understanding of the plague and its cultural-artistic consequences.

The *Triumph of Death* belongs among the early frescos in the Campo Santo, those which line the eastern arm and the eastern section of the southern arm of the cloister which shelters the monumental cemetery of the cathedral complex.[6] The fresco is part of a larger composition. On the same southern wall it is followed by the Last Judgment and the Thebaid. Our fresco elaborates, in images and accompanying texts,[7] the inexorable fact of death and decay: at the right side Death, personified as an old woman swinging her scythe, invades an orange grove sheltering unsuspecting pleasure seekers (fig. 2); at the center a cliff rises over a mound of corpses, above which angels and devils fight for the souls leaving their bodies; and at the left appears the most impressive *Meeting of the Quick and the Dead* ever painted (fig. 3). The *Thebaid* depicts the saintly lives and deaths of the anchorites of the Egyptian desert, examples of self-denial and spirituality and of man's desirable preparation for Christian death according to the dictates of faith. These panels flank the *Last Judgment* and *Hell*. Interestingly, the fear-inspiring *Inferno* is given special prominence by equalling the *Last Judgment* in scale, thus following the example of Nicola's Siena pulpit.

The frescos on the southern arm of the cloister, then, show *Man's* preoccupation *with* death. In contrast, those on the eastern arm — they originally flanked the cemetery church, the present Cappella dal Pozzo[8] — offered the Passion and Resurrection of the Lord, *His* exemplary triumph *over* Death. The *Crucifixion* appeared at the right end, facing the southern ambulatory. From technical evidence it can be shown to have been painted before the rest.[9] It was followed by the *Resurrection*, the *Witness of Christ's Wounds*, and the *Ascen-*

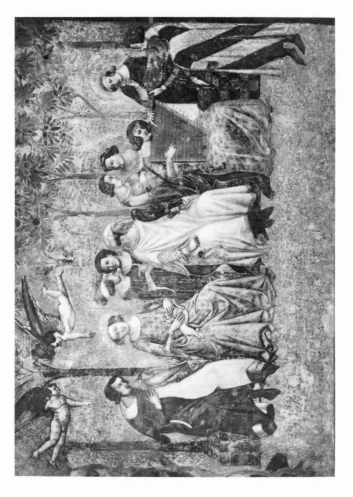

Fig. 2. Pleasure Seekers in an Orange Grove. Detail of Figure 1. (Photo Alinari)

sion, located next to the church door. These frescos, in an appropriate and effective sequence, once lined the path of the funerary procession as it proceeded from the cathedral to the church of the cemetery. No more effective monumental composition was ever devised to serve a late medieval urban cemetery than these frescos in their original locations. They are, of course, no longer *in situ*. The disastrous fire of July 1944 endangered their existence, and they were detached from their walls and relocated in the Cappella dal Pozzo and in rooms beyond the cloister of the Campo Santo. The fascinating *sinopie* which emerged beneath the frescos have now been installed in a special museum recently set up in the remodeled quarters of the Ospedale di S. Chiara, on the opposite side of the Piazza del Duomo.

The authorship of these early frescos is still debated. In recent years their Emilian origin, originally proposed by Roberto Longhi,[10] has been largely discarded. Millard Meiss gave them, except for the *Crucifixion*, to Francesco Traini.[11] Recently they have also been given to Buffalmaco.[12]

It is significant that the many texts and figures of the dead on our frescoes, as they can be discerned or as they have been transmitted by way of Renaissance copies,[13] do not refer to the plague in any way. Its symptoms are quite specific and obvious; the plague was substantially of the bubonic type, as we know from Boccaccio and other contemporary sources, causing dark swellings to develop at the neck, the armpit, the groin, sometimes as large as an egg or apple. The pneumonic plague which also raged involved coughing, a more common symptom. Since the memory of the plague had been erased by its absence from European soil over centuries, its sudden drastic return had the impact of God's wrath descending upon an unprepared and trembling Christendom.

Coeval illustrations of the Black Death have not been found, as far as I know, in Italian art. Indeed, the only direct illustration of its mortality I know of occurs in the scene of a mass burial in the annals of Gilles li Muisis, abbot of Saint Martin in Tournai, written between 1349 and 1352 (fig. 4). Specific illustrations of the plague from the Renaissance are rare. A fifteenth-century fresco from the chapel of Saint Sebastian at Lauslevillard in Savoy shows a surgeon lancing a bubo on a woman's neck.[14] Further examples remain to be discovered. By and large, the Renaissance preferred allegorical schemes that referred to the plague in terms of human fear and desired deliverance. The cult of the plague saints, especially

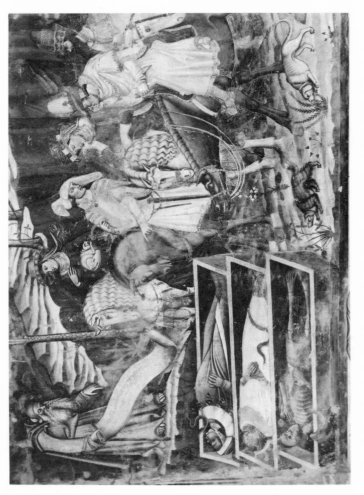

Fig. 3. Meeting of the Living and the Dead. Detail of Figure 1. (Photo Alinari)

Saint Sebastian and Saint Roch, became prominent during the later fourteenth and fifteenth centuries as a consequence of the recurrent plague epidemics.[15] The Virgin, however, more than any saint, has the power to appease God's severe judgment. Saint Sebastian had been cured by Saint Irene from the wounds of arrows with which he had been pierced by Diocletian's Mauretanian archers. The contemporary mind considered the arrow of heavenly origin to represent plague infection and mortality, a tradition reverting to antiquity; and Saint Sebastian's cure became a symbol of plague deliverance. Saint Roch's life mission was the care of the sick. He himself had contracted a severe illness which nearly cost him his life and caused a swelling to develop on his left thigh. Certainly its similarity to a pestilential bubo contributed to his popularity as a protector against the plague. However, he probably died well before the Black Death, in 1327.[16] His cult became especially pronounced in Venice, which obtained his body from his native Montpellier. Significantly, the swelling on his thigh is a constant feature of his appearance in Renaissance art.

It is useful to describe the Renaissance cult of the plague saint. Saint Roch is typically represented as looking at the swelling on his thigh, for instance in Caroto's painting in San Fermo in Verona;[17] he refers the beholder to his swelling and disease. Saint Sebastian and the Virgin, on the other hand, are endowed with the power to arrest God's pestilential arrows. Saint Sebastian thus appears on the well-known fresco in Sant' Agostino in Sant' Gimignano.[18] Here his protective mantle, held over the worshipping townspeople, stops the arrows of God's wrath. The inscription on the base supporting him asks for his intercession: "*Sancte Sebastiane intercede pro devoto populo tuo.*" This votive fresco was painted during the plague of 1464. The earliest example I know of the saint's protective mantle which arrests the heavenly arrow of disease occurs on a panel by Barnaba da Modena from the Church of the Servites in Genoa.[19] There, the *Madonna della Misericordia* protects her devotees beneath her cloak. The panel has been cut down, but enough remains to show angels with halos — they are the messengers of God's fury — who shoot arrows upon mankind. These strike all those who are not protected by the Virgin's mantle. The panel was probably painted shortly after the plague of 1372. It has been proposed that the Dominican archbishop kneeling below the Virgin is Andrea della Torre, who held office in Genoa from 1368 to 1377.[20] Barnaba da Modena resided in Genoa from 1361 to 1383. When

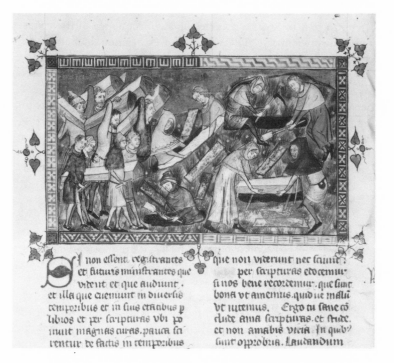

Fig. 4. Gilles li Muisis, Burial of Plague Victims in *Antiquitates Flandriae ab anno 1298 ad annum 1352.* Brussels, Bibliothèque Royale, MS no. 13076, fol. 24v. (Photo Bilbiothèque Royale)

This iconography of the saint's mantle which offers protection from the plague was first introduced remains uncertain. Of course, as was mentioned before, the arrow as harbinger of death by disease goes back to classical antiquity,[21] and the arrow as a general symbol of death appears not infrequently in early fourteenth-century Tuscan art. Francesco da Barberino, in his *Documenti d'amore*, shows Death as a four-faced figure shooting arrows from its many hands in four directions.[22] These strike their victims. Francesco's explanatory text does not refer to disease. His allegory of death returns on the funerary monument of Bishop Antonio degli Orsi by Tino di Camaino in the Cathedral of Florence, completed in 1321.[23] Jacobus de Voragine wrote of a rain of mortal arrows which fell upon Rome during the epidemic of A.D. 590.[24] When this convention was transferred to art and connected to the interceding saint is unknown. Interestingly, just a few decades separate the Genoese panel from the plague of 1348. However, the weapon of Death on

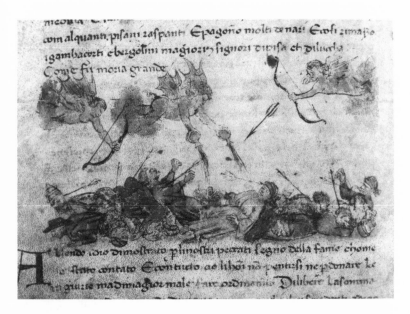

Fig. 5. Giovanni Sercambi, The Black Death of 1348 in his *Chronicle*, fol. 49v. (Photo Archivio di Stato, Lucca)

the Pisan fresco is the scythe and not the arrow.

The plague of 1348 is illustrated in the Lucchese chronicle of the apothecary Giovanni Sercambi, written around 1400 (fig. 5).[25] Corpses are piled on the ground, much like the mound of the dead on the Pisan fresco which Sercambi certainly knew. Three bat-winged demons are flying toward them, down from clouds which disclose their heavenly origin. The dead are all pierced by arrows shot by two of them, while a third empties dark liquid from two flasks. This composition is repeated in the chronicle with a few changes to illustrate other, later *trecento* epidemics like the one of 1362. We are thus observing a ritualized picture of the plague. Besides the arrows, the discharge of fluid from the vials, indicating surely the corruption of the atmosphere, would refer to the prevalent theory of *miasma*,[26] which extended from antiquity up to the nineteenth century. The most likely source for this symbolism is Apocalypse 16, in which angels pour seven vials of the wrath of God upon the earth.

We turn briefly to the north. As has been indicated, the only direct illustration of the Black Death known to me occurs in the annals of Gilles li Muisis (fig. 4). It is an example of popular realism. Artistically it does not compare with certain remarkable illuminations from the circle of Jean de Berry. Three miniatures from the *Belles Heures* by the Limbourg brothers, in the Cloisters, illustrate the institution of the great litany by Pope Gregory the Great in 590, for the purpose of combating the plague then raging in Rome.[27] The *Golden Legend* describes the elaborate procession by which Saint Gregory appeased the wrath of God, the defeat of the plague symbolized by Saint Michael standing atop the mausoleum of Hadrian (henceforth the Castel Sant' Angelo), sheathing his sword.[28] The mortality of the plague is illustrated by the dead and dying and their burial. Surprisingly, the dead seem more active than the living, one corpse falling to the ground with feet suspended in mid-air.[29] None of the dead bear the signs of the plague.

Most impressive is the double page illumination of the great procession in the *Très Riches Heures* in Chantilly, composed and begun by Pol and completed by Jean Colombe.[30] There the garments, the act of dying, and the response of the living to the sick, are all more realistic. The illustrations of the great procession of Saint Gregory seem to be additions to the original plan of these manuscripts, and certainly reflect anxiety and direct awareness of the plague or other drastic epidemic disease on the part of patron or painter, who surely had experienced them.[31]

We turn to the *Danse macabre*, the dance of the living and the dead, which subject matter captured the imagination of northern Europe during the fifteenth century and after. It has been assumed that this theme first appeared in a poem by Jean le Fèvre, dated 1376: "*Je fis de macabré la danse.*" He wrote the poem after recovery from the plague which he contracted in the epidemic that raged in Paris in 1374.[32] Thus the plague surely gave rise to the poem. Rosenfeld sees the plague of 1348 as the cause behind the earliest edition of the Latin version of the Dance of Death, which, according to him, was of German rather than French origin, having been first written by a German Dominican around 1360.[33] This is doubtful. In certain later instances the plague can be connected to the Dance of Death, as was the case of the one painted by Bernt Notke in the Marienkirche of Lübeck in 1463, just prior to the arrival of an expected plague epidemic; or the one commissioned for the Dominican cemetery in Basel in memory of the plague of 1439 which disrupted the meeting of the General Council.[34]

The most important (and probably the earliest) *danse macabre* decorated the *Cimetière des Innocents* in Paris, the central urban graveyard, sheltered inside a cloister which adjoined a Franciscan monastery. It was located in the very center of the city close to the Halles. Huizinga has aptly described the way the bustle of Parisian life spilled through its arcades, so that the mounds of skulls and the Dance of Death on the cloister walls lost their fear-inspiring awesomeness as they became familiar.[35] This *danse macabre*, a merchant writes, was begun in 1424 and completed the year after.[36] The English then occupied the city, which was, we are informed, well governed by the Duke of Bedford. The harvest happened to be good, the period a respite from recurring epidemic and the ravages of both the Hundred Years' War between the English and the French and the fighting between Armagnac and Burgundian. On the portal of the church door of the cemetery Jean de Berry had sculpted, in 1408, a *Meeting of the Quick and the Dead* which is no longer extant.[37] We recall that such a *Meeting* figures prominently in the decoration of the Pisan *Campo Santo*, and it is tempting to seek a connection.

Our brief survey of death iconography challenges the assumption of an essential link between the plague and both the *Danse macabre* and the *Meeting of the Quick and the Dead*, in the *Cimetière des Innocents*. We now return to the spectacular early frescos of the Pisan *Campo Santo* and their date. We proceed by searching for works which can be dated and which are influenced by these frescos, thus serving as *termini ante quos*.

A picture of the *Confrontation of the Living and the Dead* in the Psalter of Bonne of Luxembourg, now in the Cloisters, offers striking similarities (fig 6).[38] Following a French convention, the dead are standing, and the confrontation is distributed over two fields set on facing pages, the three dead on the right, and the three living, portrayed as equestrian hunters, on the left. The twisted neck of one horse, the pointing head of another, and the rolling eyes of all the animals show their fright. The central hunter seems to hold a sachet to his nose; he is dressed in a cloak with broad short sleeves and a *pointe-à-bec* hat. These *trois vifs* seem poorly related to these *trois morts*! The horse's stiffened neck is not oriented, as in the Pisan fresco, toward corpses lying in coffins; because the corpses are standing, the horse's position does not make sense. The central hunter's garment is real, whereas the flowing dress of his companions is purely ornamental. In addition, the landscape extending far into the

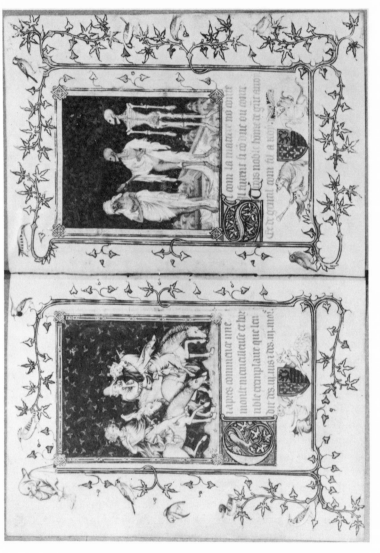

Fig. 6. Workshop of Jean Pucelle, Meeting of the Three Living and the Three Dead in the Psalter of Bonne of Luxembourg, fols. 320v–321r. Metropolitan Museum of Art, The Cloisters Collection, 1969.

distance is hardly needed by the three corpses standing on the base line of their field. The conclusion seems clear: the painter combined features taken from the Pisan fresco with themes of the French convention, not bothering to avoid inconsistencies. The psalter is close to Jean Pucelle. We recall that it was Jean Pucelle who introduced French book illumination to Italian painting — especially to Duccio. Somehow a copy of the Pisan fresco found its way into Pucelle's shop. The portrait of Bonne and her coats of arms firmly establish the psalter's ownership. It would date between her marriage in 1332 to the future John II of France and her death, by the plague, in 1349.

It stands to reason that during the turbulent period of the plague there would have been little time for painting the Pisan fresco and for its transmission beyond the Alps. The other alternative is that the Pisan fresco antedates the plague.

We now turn from *The Triumph of Death* to the fresco of *The Doubting Thomas* or *Witness of Christ's Wounds* on the eastern wall of the Campo Santo (fig. 7). Its unusual composition is also found on a relief on the funerary monument of Cardinal Luca Fieschi in the Cathedral of Genoa (fig. 8). The oblong relief extends over three squarish stone plates. Christ is surrounded by the Apostles. In the center plate a frontal Christ reveals the *stigmata*. Five Apostles hold his arms, point toward his wounds, kiss them, talk about them. This composition duplicates much of the Pisan fresco, and in both Christ wears a cope with an ornate border clasped by a brooch.

It would be better to title the relief *The Apostles' Adoration of the Stigmata*. This subject matter had a currency limited to the *trecento* which included, besides the Genoese relief and the Pisan fresco, a painting by Bartolo di Fredi in Pienza, a late *trecento* fresco near Florence, a painting by Taddeo Gaddi in the Accademia, and an interesting fresco, dated 1338 by inscription, in the Duomo of Pistoia, attributed recently to Giovanni di Bartolommeo Cristiani.[39]

The Pisan fresco is half destroyed, but enough remains to show that it preceded the Genoese relief. The latter is so similar to the former that the one work is obviously copied from the other, even to the pattern of folds around the feet of the stooping apostle. The compositions vary, however, in one important element. On the Pisan fresco the apostles are closely packed about Christ, forming a V-shape which recurs on the later fresco in Pistoia. On the Genoese relief, though, the figures are densely packed only on the central slab, to the sides of which they are loosely spaced. Nor is the work-

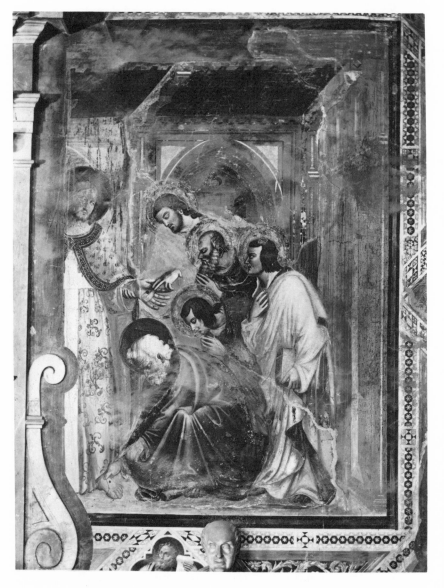

Fig. 7. Francesco Traini, The Apostles' Witness of the Stigmata. Pisa, Campo Santo. (Photo Alinari)

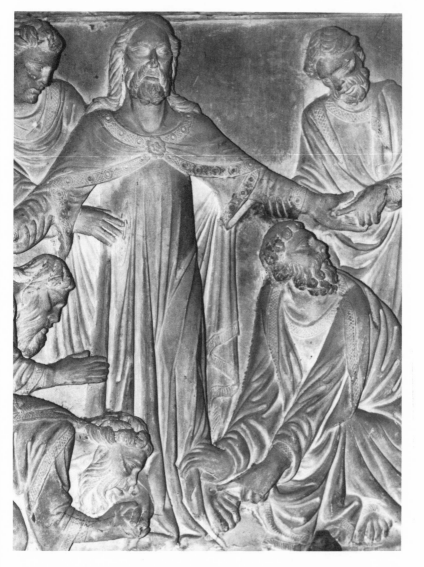

Fig. 8. The Apostles' Witness of the Stigmata. Relief from the tomb of Luca Fieschi, Cathedral of Genoa. (Photo by Polzer)

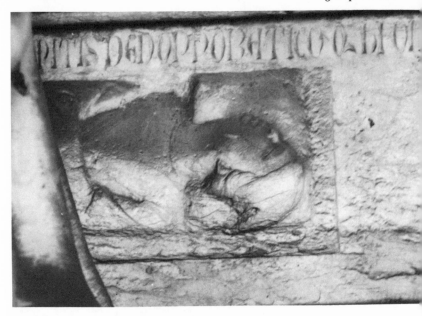

Fig. 9. Funerary Relief of Gherardo della Gherardesca.
Pisa, Campo Santo. (Photo by Polzer)

manship — by a Pisan-trained traveling sculptor — of high quality.
He quoted a fresco with which he was familiar.

Luca Fieschi died in 1336. Documents inform us that his tomb
was not quite completed in 1342.[40] By that time the *Passion of Christ*
in the Campo Santo already existed.

Further information is found in the Campo Santo itself. The
funeral monument of the Gherardesca, a most prominent family
whose members ruled Pisa during a good part of the first half of
the *trecento*, has been relocated in the Campo Santo from San
Francesco, its original site. It was probably erected shortly after
the death of Gaddo Gherardesca in 1320. To it was added the sar-
cophagus of Gherardo (fig. 9), the son of Bonifazio Novello, Lord
of Pisa from 1330 to 1340. An inscription informs us that the boy
died in 1336. He is shown in shallow relief on the front of the sar-
cophagus, lying on his back with hands crossed over the torso: the
normal position of sculptures of the deceased. His head is thrown
back in sharp profile so that it tilts down from the neck. This feature
is exceptional for its period when the sculpted deceased rested their
heads on pillows. It anticipates the relaxed heads of later *transis* —
witness Pilon's *Henry II* from his tomb at Saint Denis.[41] Possibly,

this exceptionally informal effigy was commissioned by an extremely devout and humble father, who in his own will insisted that his own death not be commemorated in any way.

This unusually angled head would seem to copy the coffined corpses of the Pisan *Triumph of Death*, or those heaped at the center of the fresco. This would mean that the fresco was already done by 1336.

It is possible that the fresco was quoted in an even earlier relief: *Christ Curing the Lame* from Andrea's door on the Baptistery in Florence (fig. 10). It was completed in 1336, but the models, preparatory to casting, must have been finished some years before, probably before the drastic flood of 1333. The two cripples imploring Christ's assistance are quite similar to the two extreme figures in the Pisan work of the lame and sick clamoring for the release of death (fig. 11). Situated close to the base line of the fresco, they would have been easily observable by Andrea. In addition, the disciple of John the Baptist behind the two cripples on the bronze panel is similar to a bearded oriental in the bottom tier of the damned in the Pisan *Last Judgment*.[42] Examples can be extended.

The Campo Santo frescos were painted before the Black Death of 1348. They were surely completed before 1333–1336. This chronology connects directly with the one presented in the *Art Bulletin* of 1964.[43] I discussed there the anti-Ghibelline propaganda of these frescos which links them to Pisan history of the late thirteen-twenties. Vasari identified in the *Triumph of Death*, among the hunters and in the orange grove, the Ghibelline captains Uguccione della Faggiola and Castruccio, and the German emperor Ludwig the Bavarian. This excommunicated emperor was in Pisa in 1328, at the climax of his conflict with Pope John XXII. He was accompanied by his antipope, Nicholas V, the Franciscan Pietro da Corvara. The latter is probably depicted among the schismatics cut to pieces by demons. He is tonsured and named by inscription "Nicolò, Lover of Mohammed." Mohammed himself, according to Dante the archetype of the schismatics, is depicted below Nicolò. He is throttled, and Antichrist is flayed beside him. The frescos in the Campo Santo belong to the years after Ludwig's Pisan episode and before the completion of Andrea's Florentine doors — that is, the first years of the thirties. The frescos thus had nothing to do with the plague.

Death is a perpetual human dilemma. An intensifying preoccupation with natural death and decay is evident in the later Mid-

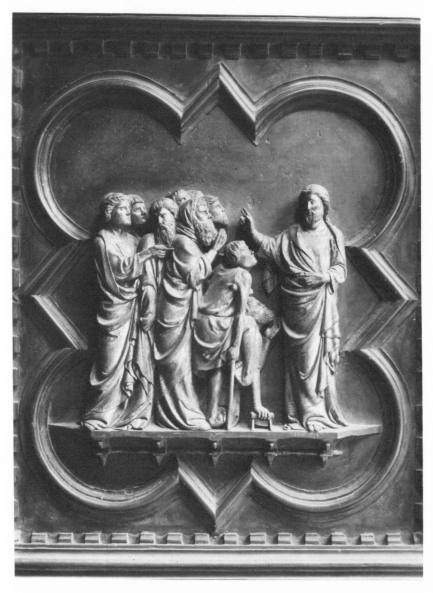

Fig. 10. Andrea Pisano, Christ Healing the Lame.
Florence, the Baptistery, bronze door. (Photo Brogi)

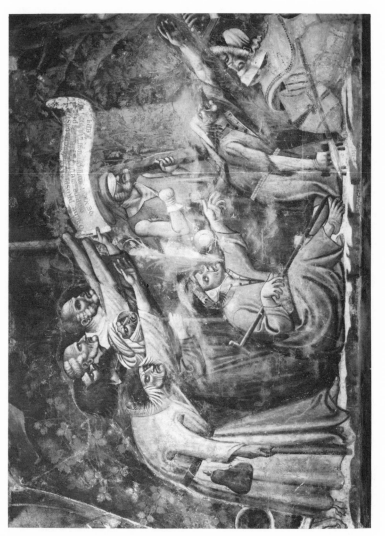

Fig. 11. The Sick and Lame Yearning for Death. Detail of Figure 1. (Photo Alinari)

dle Ages. This intensified concern with natural death can be considered a by-product of a remarkable late medieval prosperity which gave rise to the growth of the towns and the democratization of religious devotion. Monumental urban cemeteries were then prepared to collect the dead and cleanse important civic precincts of graves in the path of ordered urban growth. These cemeteries were given the shape of cloisters; they were attached to funerary chapels or churches; and they were given decoration to suit their function. The same would hold true of hospitals. The hospital set up in Palermo in the Palazzo Sclafani, after 1435, was decorated with a remarkable *Triumph of Death*, situated in the court, probably during the early 1440s, by an unknown artist.[44] An equestrian, skeletal Death slays his victims with his arrows. The victims do not show plague symptoms; however, the plague ravaged Barcelona during the years 1439–1441, and it might have reached Palermo. It is significant that certain features of the fresco clearly betray an awareness of the Pisan *Triumph of Death*.

The disruptive power of the great pandemic of 1348, destroying suddenly one-third to one-fourth of the population of western Europe, created conditions of chaos and social disruption so severe that they certainly terminated significant artistic production of any kind while the plague raged. Only retrospectively did man assess this extreme catastrophe in artistic and literary terms, as did Boccaccio in his *Decameron*. This assessment could make use of precedent only in a limited way, for the Black Death struck as something entirely new and unpredictable, since its earlier European presence had been erased from memory by an absence of six centuries. As the plague returned periodically after the Black Death with lessened epidemic intensity, a plague iconography gradually evolved reflecting the personal and collective yearning for protection. However, it must be kept in mind that dying is a constant human concern which does not wait for epidemics. Accordingly, the Pisan *Triumph of Death*, the most spectacular representation of this subject matter from the Middle Ages or the Renaissance, has nothing to do with the plague, which it precedes by nearly two decades. Instead, it offers a brutally direct monumental *memento mori* to a prosperous community, a perpetual reminder that in the Christian scheme death is a condition necessary for obtaining ultimate grace and eternal life.

notes

1. Millard Meiss, *Painting in Florence and Siena after the Black Death* (Princeton, 1951), p. 74.

2. Frederick Hartt, *A History of Italian Renaissance Art*, 3rd ed. (Englewood, N.J., 1975), p. 102.

3. Hellmut Rosenfeld, *Der mittelalterliche Totentanz: Entstehung, Entwicklung, Bedeutung*, 3rd ed. (Cologne-Vienna, 1974), p. 172. See also Liliane Brion-Guerry, *Le thème du "Triomphe de la Mort" dans la peinture italienne* (Paris, 1950), p. 130.

4. Robert Oertel, *Early Italian Painting to 1400* (New York, 1968), 305 ff.

5. Joseph Polzer, "Aristotle, Mohammed and Nicholas V in Hell," *Art Bulletin* 46 (1964): 457–69, especially pp. 467–69. I presented further evidence for an early dating in a paper presented to the College Art Association in Chicago in January 1971; see also Florens Deuchler, "Looking at Bonne of Luxembourg's Prayer Book," *Metropolitan Museum of Art Bulletin* 29 (1971): 267–78, especially 267; Millard Meiss, "Notable Disturbances in the Classification of Tuscan Trecento Paintings," *The Burlington Magazine* 113 (1971): 171–86, especially 181; Hanns Swarzenski, "Before and After Pisano," *Boston Museum Bulletin* 68 (1970): 178–96, especially 194–95; Luciano Bellosi, *Buffalmacco e il Trionfo della Morte* (Turin, 1974), 41 ff.; Polzer, below, n. 39. I am presently examining the chronological location of these frescos within the later 20's or early 30's.

6. For reproductions of the early frescos in the Campo Santo in Pisa see Mario Bucci and Licia Bertolini, *Camposanto monumentale di Pisa: Affreschi e sinopie* (Pisa, 1960); also Millard Meiss, "The Problem of Francesco Traini," *Art Bulletin* 15 (1933): 97–173.

7. S. Morpurgo, "Le epigrafi volgari in rima del Trionfo della Morte," *L'Arte* 2 (1899): 51 ff.

8. A text located on the first pilaster at the right side of the facade of Pisa Cathedral, dated 1299 (1300 *stile Pisano*) records that Borgundio di Tado, *operaio* from 1298 to 1311, "fecie fare l'eclesia di chanpo sancto dall'ar-coara in su." Three other documents of the same year refer to its interior decoration (given by Tanfani Centofanti in *Notizie di artisti e tratti dai documenti pisani* (Pisa, 1897), 492 f. There can be little doubt that the church of the Campo Santo is identical with the present Cappella dal Pozzo. This chapel forms the head of the entire monumental cemetery, located off the center of the elevated eastern cloister arm. Aspects of its marble revetment, visible from the exterior, indicate that it was part of the original building program. But see A. Caleca, *Pisa-Museo delle Sinopie del Camposanto Monumentale* (Pisa, 1979), p. 43, where he locates this church on the second story of the house containing the *Opera della Primaziale*.

9. The remains of the *sottostrapo* still *in situ* on the wall of the *Crucifixion* fresco adjoining the southeastern corner of the cloister and the wall bearing the *Triumph of Death* show clearly, by the overlay of the respective wall surfaces, that the *Crucifixion* preceded the *Triumph of Death*; see also the article by Millard Meiss cited in n. 5 above, p. 182, n. 15, giving infor-

mation obtained from Leonetto Tintori.

10. "Vitale da Bologna e i suoi affreschi nel Camposanto di Pisa," *Mitteilungen des Kunsthistorischen Instituts in Florenz* 4 (1933): 135–37; more recently, Enzo Carli, *Pittura medievale pisana* (Milan, 1958), 1:58 ff., considers that Traini was replaced by an Emilian painter in the Thebaid.

11. See the Meiss articles cited in nn. 5 and 6 above.

12. See the Bellosi book cited in n. 5 above.

13. *Cf.* the article by Morpurgo, n. 7 above.

14. Reproduced in Jean-Noël Biraben, *Les hommes et la peste en France et dans les pays européens et mediterranéens* (Paris, 1976), 2:fig. 5.

15. Raymond Henry Payne Crawfurd, *Plague and Pestilence in Literature and Art* (Oxford, 1914), passim. See also, recently, H. H. Mollaret and J. Brossolet, "La peste, source méconnue d'inspiration artistique," *Koninklijk Museum voor schone Kunsten, Antwerpen, Jaarboek* (1965), pp. 3–112 for an interesting compilation of plague-related pictures.

16. The accounts of the life of Saint Roch place him into the beginning and also into the second half of the fourteenth century (see *Acta Sanctorum, augusti iii*, 380 ff.; *Lexikon der christlichen Ikonographie*, VIII (1975), 275 f.; J. Cambell in the *New Catholic Encyclopedia*, XII (1966), 540 f. — favoring the later chronology).

17. Crawfurd, plate XII, passim. The cult of Saint Roch flourished from the late quattrocento onward.

18. Reproduced in Crawfurd, plate VII.

19. Reproduced in P. Rotondi, *La madonna nell'arte in Liguria: Dipinti e sculture dal secolo XIII al XVIII* (catalogue of the exhibition in the Palazzo dell'Accademia, 30 April-31 May 1952), plates 3–5 and p. 16, n. 4.

20. Mario Labo dates the panel shortly after 1372 in G. B. Bono and Mario Labo, *Nostra Signora dei Servi* (Genoa, 1927), pp. 34–35.

21. *Iliad* I, 1 ff.; Deut. 32:23.

22. Reproduced in Bernhard Degenhart and Annegrit Schmitt, *Corpus der italienischen Zeichnungen, 1300–1450* (Berlin, 1968), vol. 1, pt. 1, figs. 50 and 63.

23. Reproduced in R. W. Valentiner, *Tino di Camaino, A Sienese Sculptor of the Fourteenth Century* (Paris, 1935), plates 27 and 28.

24. Jacobus de Voragine, *The Golden Legend*, trans. Granger Ryan and Helmut Ripperger (1941; reprint ed., New York, 1969), p. 179.

25. Salvatore Bongi, ed., *Le chroniche di Giovanni Sercambi*, 3 vols. (Lucca, 1892), vol. 1:96.

26. Leonard Fabian Hirst, *The Conquest of Plague: A Study of the Evolution of Epidemiology* (Oxford, 1953), 35 ff. A flying angel pouring corrupted air from two vessels appears in Mignard's lost *Plague of David*, of which an engraved copy is reproduced in Crawfurd, plate III.

27. Reproduced in Millard Meiss, *French Painting in the Time of Jean de Berry: The Limbourgs and their Contemporaries*, vol. 2, *Plates* (New York, 1974), figs. 451, 452, 641.

28. Translation cited in n. 24, p. 180.

29. Meiss as cited in n. 27, fig. 641.

30. Ibid., figs. 575 and 576.

31. The *Chronique du Religieux de Saint Denis* (Paris, 1840), 2:692–93, describes an intense epidemic which ravaged the area around Paris from 1399 to 1402. According to Meiss's recent persuasive discussion of its chronology (cited in n. 27:vol. 1, *Text*, p. 103), the Belles Heures were painted in 1408, the same year in which Jean de Berry had the relief of the Meeting of the Three Living and Three Dead carved for the portal of the Church of the Innocents, according to a lost inscription (see below, n. 37). Both the relief and the illustrations of the plague of Saint Gregory in the Belles Heures would document the duke's awareness of death, which was surely accentuated by the disease from which he barely recovered, contracted during a violent epidemic in the spring of 1404.

32. Rosenfeld, cited above, n. 3, 123 f.

33. Ibid., 64 ff., especially p. 71.

34. Ibid., p. 183; the Basel *Danse macabre* no longer exists, but it was copied by Mérion in 1621, who gave the following explanation: "Ce tableau est un vieux monument et une rare antiquité qui y fut fondée par le grand concile, par les pères et les prélats qui y assistaient des temps de l'Empereur Sigismond en mémoire perpétuelle de la mortalité ou de la peste qui y regnait en 1439 pendant le Concile" (after J. Brossolet, *Les danses macabres en temps de peste: Koninklijk Museum voor schone Kunsten, Antwerpen, Jaarboek* [1971], pp. 43–44).

35. Johan Huizinga, *The Waning of the Middle Ages* (New York, 1967), 130 ff., esp. 133 ff.

36. Alexandre Tuetey, ed., *Journal d'un bourgeois de Paris, 1405–1449* (Paris, 1881), p. 203.

37. Karl Künstle, *Die Legende der drei Lebenden und der drei Toten und der Totentanz* (Freiburg im Breisgau, 1908), p. 57 (after Jacques de Breul, *Le théâtre d'antiquitez de Paris* [1642], p. 834), quotes the inscription which accompanied the portal relief:

> En l'an mil quatre cents et huict,
> Jean duc de Berry tres puissant,
> Fit tailler ici sa sepulture
> Des trois vifs assi des trois morts.

The date of 1408 conflicts with the fact that by 1405 Jean de Berry had dedicated his intended funerary shrine, the Sainte Chapelle in Bourges.

38. And see the article of Deuchler cited in n. 5 above.

39. Miklos Boskovits, "Un'opera probabile di Giovanni di Bartolomeo Cristiani e l'iconografia della 'preparazione alla crocifissione'," *Acta Historiae Artium* (Academia Scientiarum Hungarica) 11 (1965): 69–94; also Joseph Polzer, "Christ Judge, Saviour, Advocate, Franciscan Devotion, and the Doubting Thomas," *Essays Presented to Myron P. Gilmore* (Florence, 1978), 2:301–10.

40. For the documents concerning the erection of the Luca Fieschi tomb, see Federigo Alizeri, *Notizie de'professori del disegno in Liguria* (Genoa, 1870-80), 5:40; also D. G. Salvi, *La cattedrale di Genova* (1931), p. 1001, n. 56.

41. Reproduced in Horst Woldemar Janson, *History of Art* (New York, 1969), p. 404 fig. 602.

42. Reproduced in Bucci and Bertolini, as cited in n. 6 above, Plate XV. Other paintings preceding the Black Death of 1348 which are influenced by the Pisan *Triumph of Death* include the *Meeting of the Living and the Dead* by Jacopo del Casentino in the collection of the University of Göttingen, dated by Richard Offner in the painter's middle period (*A Critical and Historical Corpus of Florentine Painting*, sec. 5, vol. 2, pt. 2, plate LI no. 2, p. 128), also in *Bolletino d'Arte* 3 (1923): 248-84, at p. 281, and by Wolfgang Stechow in the fourth decade of the *trecento: Zeitschrift für bildende Kunst* 48 (1924-25): 210; the *predella* panels of the *Meeting of the Living and the Dead*, attributed to an assistant of Bernardo Daddi, in the Accademia in Florence, placed by Offner in the early forties (op. cit. sec. 3, vol. 5, pp. 81-82, plate XVI no. 3-4); and the illumination of the same subject in a hymnal in the Biblioteca Nazionale in Florence, the Laudario Magliabechiano, formerly no. II, I, 122, new catalogue no. BR 18, fol. 134r, which has been linked to the circle of Pacino da Buonaguida or the Lorenzetti and placed in the thirties: Fernando Liuzzi, *La lauda e i primordi della melodia italiana* (Rome, 1933), 1:77-81; Paolo d'Ancona, *La miniatura fiorentina* (1914), 2:94; Mario Salmi in *La Bibliofilia* 33 (1932): 273 ff.

43. Cited in n. 5 above.

44. Maria Grazia Paolini, "Il Trionfo della Morte di Palermo e la cultura internazionale", *Rivista dell'Istituto Nazionale di Archeologia e Storia dell'Arte*, n.s. 11-12 (1963), pp. 301-69, precisely at 302-3, refers to papers uncovered behind that fresco when it was removed from the wall, bearing the date 1441. Recently, Jane Bridgeman has placed the fresco in the period 1438-45 on the basis of the fashions in clothing: "The Palermo Triumph of Death", *Burlington Magazine* 117 (1975): 480-484. The close iconographic link of the Palermitan *Triumph of Death* with those of the Pisan Campo Santo and Lorenzetti's in the Pinacoteca in Siena has been often underscored. Different from the latter, however, the Palermitan fresco shows all the dead and dying pierced by arrows. Given the widespread use of the arrow as a symbol of plague contagion during the quattrocento, the question arises whether a traditional Triumph of Death has here been adapted to the depiction of epidemic disease. 1441 witnessed an intense plague in Barcelona, which may also have reached Palermo (for the plague in Barcelona, see Biraben, as in n. 14 above, vol. 1, p. 216). A mound of dead, killed by the Black Death, each pierced by an arrow, appears already in Sercambi's illustration of the great epidemic of 1348 (fig. 5), and on a plague banner by Bonfigli (reproduced in Crawfurd, as cited in n. 15 above, Plate XIV). A skeletal, bat-winged Death stands beneath a monumental *Madonna della Misericordia*, shooting arrows indiscriminately upon the townspeople.

Pestilence and
Middle English Literature:
Friar John Grimestone's
Poems on Death

Siegfried Wenzel

The Black Death: a fatal epidemic sweeping through most of the civilized world; striking suddenly and killing young and old, rich and poor, saint and sinner; filling houses and streets with corpses that had to be hastily buried, often in huge pits without the rites and decorum of a proper funeral; and leaving behind it stunned men and women bereft of relatives, friends, and neighbors, desolated villages, and the threats of economic, social, and moral disaster. How is this cataclysmic event reflected in the poetry of the survivors?

In examining the impact of the plague on Middle English literature, we should first remind ourselves that the name "Black Death," denoting the great bubonic epidemic of 1348–49, began to be used only in the nineteenth century. Medieval writers in English referred to the plague simply as "pestilence" or "death" with at best such qualifiers as "foul," "great," or "first." Linguistic usage here neatly reflects history: the Black Death of 1348 was only the first of a long series of major epidemics occurring in England and Europe with varying degrees of intensity and spreading over more than three centuries. Hence it may be advisable to broaden our interest in the Black Death and ask how the experience of the Great Plague and its successors is reflected in late medieval literature. Nonetheless, in keeping with the theme of this conference I will focus on English documents that were written during the first half century after the Black Death, that is, up until approximately 1400.

Apart from chronicles and medical or astrological treatises, the literature of this period contains surprisingly few references to the plague, and the few which do occur are usually remarks made in passing. In vain does one look for a parallel from an English quill

to the long and moving descriptions of the Black Death given by
Boccaccio[1] and by Machaut,[2] or to the anguished outcry in one
of Petrarch's letters.[3] In the Canterbury Tales Chaucer uses the
word *pestilence* nine times; but on three occasions it merely means
"the highest degree of" some moral evil,[4] and three other passages
use it in the formula of a curse, such as the Wife of Bath's farewell
benediction:

> And olde and angry nygardes of dispence,
> God sende hem soone verray pestilence![5]

Chaucer's contemporary, William Langland, refers just as many
times to the pestilence, but in contrast to Chaucer, his allusions,
brief as they are, vibrate with historical relevance and emotional
intensity. Three of them speak of various kinds of moral deteriora-
tion that have occurred "since pestilence time": priests have left their
parishes because of their congregations' poverty;[6] marriages made
since the plague are without love;[7] and friars "sithe the pestilences"
have been inventing and debating far-fetched theological questions
and have been preaching "at saint Poules" "in pure enuye of clerkes"
instead of strengthening the people's faith and leading them to re-
pentance.[8] A more legitimate kind of preaching is pictured in the
long discourse of Reason who, among many other things, "prouede
that thuse pestilences / Was for pure synne, to punysche the pu-
ple."[9] Together with other natural disasters pestilence is again mentioned in a warning to all men to work while it is time or else hunger
will return and the following fate will befall:

> Through floods and foul weather shall harvests fail,
> Pride and pestilences shall fetch many people.[10]

Such a warning forecast is turned into an almost apocalyptic vision near the end of the poem when the poet's sight focuses on Antichrist's attack on Unity. As more and more people gather behind
Antichrist's banner, Conscience calls Nature in for help, and the
latter, together with Old Age and Death, unleashes sicknesses and
plagues as a clear signal to wicked men to amend their evil lives:

> Hoar Old Age was in the vanguard
> And bore the banner before Death, he claimed it as
> > his right.

Nature followed him with many kinds of sores,
Such as pocks and pestilences, and she harmed many
                                                  people;
So Nature killed many through corruptions.
Death came driving after her and dashed all to dust,
Kings and knights, emperors and popes;
He left no man standing, whether learned or ignorant;
Whatever he hit stirred never afterwards.
Many a lovely lady and their lover-knights
Swooned and died in sorrow of Death's blows.[11]

This short paragraph of alliterative verse is the most brilliant poetic expression of the plague experience that remains from medieval England. It is also quite typical of the emotional and intellectual reaction to the plague as Langland and his contemporaries experienced it: together with other natural disasters the plague is an instance of divine action, carried out through natural agents, to punish evildoers but also — and more prominently so — to call erring mankind back from their wicked ways. In two further passages Langland reflects on man's helplessness in the face of these disasters. The first states that "prayers have no power to prevent these pestilences":

For God is deaf nowadays and will not hear us,
And for our guilt he grinds good men to dust.[12]

The second alludes to the promise Christ gave his apostles that they would heal sickness and then notes that the promise does not work for the present-day pope, who is unable "to stop this unhealthy air and to heal the sick." But Langland excuses the pope and instead blames the people's failure to effect moral improvement in their own conduct:

But if the power to work miracles fails him, it is
                                because men are not worthy
To have God's grace, and there is no fault in the
                                                  pope.
For no blessing can do us good unless we correct
                                                  ourselves.[13]

Similarly, the deafness of God to men's prayers that was spoken of in the first passage is seen as a consequence of pride in all strata of society, particularly in the frivolous and pointless preaching of the friars which we heard of earlier; God grinds good men to death "for *oure* gultes."

Langland's statements about *pestilence* parallel the various forms and sentiments of the sporadic references to the plague which I have been able to find in other English writings up to the beginning of the fifteenth century. The formula "since pestilence time" appears again, almost as a tag, in *Mum and the Sothsegger*, [14] and a handful of texts list the plague with other disasters as "warnings and tokens that God sends us everyday."[15] Of slightly greater interest is the prose treatise *Dives and Pauper*, a lengthy exposition of the Ten Commandments in dialogue form.[16] It mentions the plague, here called *moreyn*, several times, always in conjunction with other natural disasters, and asks whether these are caused by the stars and may therefore be foreseen by astrological inquiry. The answer is solidly orthodox and very skeptical about planetary causation: God is above the stars and may use other agents — including good and evil angels — to chastise men for their sins and to show his might;[17] hence the stars may foretell a disaster but are not reliable, and experience has shown that plagues strike "sometimes in one town and not in another; sometimes on one side of the street and not on the other," even though the evil star did in fact pass over both.[18] Consequently it is great folly for men to postpone moral reform until they are warned of possible death by astrology or other forms of divination;[19] it is similarly foolish "to trust in these fasts that have been recently instituted to escape sudden death" because God will not be tied down by human machinations.[20] As one can infer from these references, all mentions of the plague in *Dives and Pauper* occur in the section on the First Commandment which is devoted to the discussion of various superstitions.

At this point our inquiry may well come to a halt for lack of fuel, because explicit references to the plague in devotional and instructional works, and even more so in imaginative literature, are scarce in number and meager in content. To pursue the question of how the medieval plague experience is reflected in literature further, I propose to turn to Middle English lyrics that deal with the topic of death and to see whether and in what ways their representation of death and reaction to it changed after the Black Death. Lyrics are the best literary genre for such a test because the vast majority of them produced in the fourteenth century is intimately connected with the same context from which the already surveyed references to the plague had come, that is, religio-moral instruction and particularly preaching. From Chaucer's Pardoner to Langland's friars, Reason, and the visionary poet himself, and beyond to a manual on the Decalogue, our best passages have had something to do with sermons and religious instruction. Just so, fourteenth-century lyrics on death are vitally related to contemporary preaching, because most of them were made for and used in sermons, and their majority has been preserved in manuscripts that collect either complete sermons or commonplace material which preachers would have used in their ministry.[21]

I am referring to the so-called "preachers' tags": mostly rather short English poems that are found in the body of sermons which, before 1400, were still written down in Latin. They serve a variety of functions: some versify the main division of a sermon, others sum up the moral of a sermon story, and still others render in English a biblical proof-text or some other "authority." Many were used to help preachers and their audiences remember some essential points, but others served more as punch lines, and quite a number of them even reveal some delight in punning and in "wit."[22] The largest body of such verses made during the half century following the Black Death appears in the Commonplace Book written by Friar John Grimestone in 1372.[23] In one hundred and forty sections[24] arranged alphabetically it gathers commonplace material which he and presumably his fellow preachers would use in treating such sermon topics as abstinence, confession, Christ's passion, prayer, truth, and a host of others including death. The material includes many quotations from the Bible, the Church Fathers and more recent theologians, and classical authors; topics and schemata of current popular preaching; an occasional story in shortened form; and a large number of verses and proverbs in Latin, French, and English. Of English verses Grimestone's book contains a total of 246.[25]

In order to compare Grimestone's verses with similar poems written before the Black Death, I choose the *Fasciculus morum*, a discursive treatment of the seven deadly sins and related matters made shortly after the year 1300 by a Franciscan author for the use of his fellow preachers.[26] Like Grimestone's Commonplace Book, *Fasciculus morum* weaves together a large number of biblical, patristic, and classical "authorities," of *distinctiones* and schemata, of similes and sermon stories (here often followed by long moralizations), and of Latin and English preachers' verses. Of the latter there are fifty-five in the handbook, and six of them appear in a single chapter devoted to meditation on death. This chapter deserves closer attention because it gathers up the commonplace thoughts as well as rhetorical devices that had become standard in popular preaching on death by the beginning of the fourteenth century.

The chapter in question appears in the section devoted to pride. Among several considerations which may lead man to the opposite virtue, humility, the second is this:

> keep death in mind, for as Jerome says: "He who considers himself as about to die easily scorns all things." And according to the counsel of the wise man: "Remember thy last end and thou shalt never sin" [Ecclesiasticus 7.40]. Whence it is said in a verse:

> > Non aliter poterit melius caro viva domari,
> > Mortua qualis erit quam semper premeditari.

Which in English is as follows:

> > þe flesches lust may þou nouȝt o-lyue bettur quenche,
> > Bot aftur þy deth which þou beȝ euermore beþenche,

[You cannot quench carnal lust any better in this life than by always reflecting on what you will be after your death]

that is to say, how short and uncertain life is and how vile our dead body. According to Job, "Man born of woman," and so forth. In English:

> > Mon iboren of wommon ne lyueth but a stounde,
> > In wrechednes and in wo ben his dayes iwounde.
> > He springus out as blossome and sone falles to grounde,
> > And wendes away as schadewe þat no wey is ifounde.

[Man born of woman lives for only an hour; his days are wrapped in wretchedness and woe. He bursts forth like a blossom, but soon falls to the ground, and he passes away like a shadow that is nowhere found.]

For he lives in much labor and ends in pain. And whatever was lovable to men in life will be hateful and abominable to them in death. Just as a candle when it is blown out does not serve those who are present, but certainly that which used to comfort people smells most badly — just so is it with man when he dies, for his body, which in life used to comfort many, becomes to them an object of horror in death. According to those verses:

> Vilior est humana caro quam pellis ovina:
> Cum moritur ovis aliquid valet illa ruina,
> Extrahitur pellis et scribitur intus et extra;
> Cum moritur homo moritur simul caro et ossa.

[Man's flesh is more worthless than sheepskin. When a sheep dies, its demise is of some value, for its skin is taken off and written upon on both sides. But when man dies, both his flesh and bones are gone.]

Therefore St. Bernard says: "When a man dies, his nose grows cold, his face turns white, his nerves and veins break, his heart splits in two. Nothing is more horrible than his corpse: it is not left in the house lest the family should die; it is not thrown into water lest it should cause infection; it is not hung up in the air lest it should corrupt it; but like pestilential poison it is thrown into a pit so that it may no longer be seen; it is surrounded with earth so that its stench cannot rise; it is firmly stamped down so that it may not rise again, but rather that earth may remain in earth and man's eyes may no longer behold it." Therefore it is said in English:

> Was þer neuer caren so lothe
> As mon when he to put goth
>   And deth has layde so lowe.
> For when deth drawes mon from oþur,
> Pe suster nul not se þe brother,
>   Ne fader þe sone i-knawe.

[Never was there such loathsome carrion as when man goes to the pit and death has laid him so low. For when death separates man from his fellow, a sister does not want to see her brother, nor a father know his son.]

And Bede says that remembering death makes humility win out. Therefore let us think upon the shortness of time, the certainty of death, and the fickleness of our friends, and let us always be prepared, because indeed our day is most certain, even if altogether unknown. We do not know if it comes at midnight, or at the cock's crow, or in the morning, for man is taken away from our midst "like the shadow when it declineth" [cf. Psalm 108.23]; and "as a ship that passeth through the waves, wherof when it is gone by, the trace cannot be found" [Wisdom 5.10], "so we also being born forthwith have ceased to be" [Wisdom 5.13]. Since death is common to all, it is said that one and the same captivity will overcome all. Whence it is told that Alexander in a letter asked his teacher Aristotle four questions. . . .

These questions are all of the type "What is it that the longer and higher it grows, the shorter and smaller it becomes?" and deal with life, the corpse, the dead man's friends, and his possessions which are distributed among his executors, where those riches can do his soul no good. This point leads our preacher into another brief tale about a cleric in Paris who had a tomb sculpted for himself with an image that would always remind him of his own death and of his indifferent executors. The tomb bears inscriptions of French and English verses. Then the author proposes an acrostic on the Latin word M-O-R-S, by which death is likened to a mirror, a clock, a thief, and a summoner. Each property of death is developed at some length. The following lines will indicate the richness and vitality of the imagery that is here gathered:

Death is likened to a clock, whose function is to waken religious people to pray. But lazy folk, after hearing the first stroke, wait for the second, and often they are so heavy with sleep that they do not hear it. . . . Clocks have different songs. The song of this clock is, "Remember thy last end, and thou shalt never sin." In English:

> Haue mynde on þyn ende,
> And euer fro synne þou myght wende.

. . . Finally, Death is likened to a summoner. As the summoner carries letters or a rod as a sign of his office, thus Death instead of a rod carries an arrow of the sharpest pain. Hence according to the ancients Death was depicted as a knight on horseback carrying a square shield, in whose first quartering was an ape grinning, indicating that after death a man's executors laugh at him and spend his goods after their pleasure. In the second quartering was painted a lion raging, for just as a lion when he catches his prey utters a terrible cry at which the other animals stand still so that the lion can go around and catch them as he pleases—just so Death halts all around him and devours them as he wants. In the third quartering was an archer, showing that the last blow man will bear is death. And in the fourth quartering was a scribe, indicating that all our deeds will be written down and recited before God, the good as well as the evil ones, after man's death. This summoner Death first summons us to death in youth, next he binds us to appear in court, in the strength of adolescence, thirdly he imprisons us in old age through our natural weaknesses, and finally after the verdict of the jury before God our judge we will be given life or death as we have deserved. "O death, how bitter is the remembrance of thee!" [Ecclesiasticus 41.1].[27]

From this earlier exhortation to meditate on death we now turn to Grimestone's verses written over two generations later but at a time when the memory of the Black Death presumably was still very fresh. Grimestone's section *De morte*[28] comprises twenty-two English poems,[29] and to these I would add six more found in other sections but also dealing explicitly with death.[30] A group of twenty-eight poems may at first sight appear as an impressively large collection of verses on this topic, but this percentage diminishes in impressiveness when we realize that these are twenty-eight out of 246 verses. In contrast, *Fasciculus morum* offers a total of thirteen poems dealing with death out of fifty-five English verses in the handbook.[31] If numbers alone can tell us anything, it would seem that the preoccupation with death was considerably greater in the earlier work; the plague experience of 1348 certainly had no discernible effect on the output of death lyrics. The same inference can be drawn from comparing the two groups of poems with respect to their size. Grimestone's poems are quite short. Half of them consist of two rhyming couplets each, another eight are only single couplets, and only two poems reach as many as twelve and sixteen lines respectively. This brevity is quite in keeping with pre-Black

Death traditions, and throughout the fourteenth century most preachers' verses on death remained very short.

A similar continuity shows in the relation of these poems to their sources and backgrounds. A large percentage of English preachers' verses on any topic were directly translated from Latin models, either prose passages or verses. In medieval sermon collections and handbooks for preachers written in Latin, the Latin model usually is given first and then rendered into vernacular rhymes, a technique illustrated by the *Fasciculus morum* passage which was quoted earlier. All these characteristics apply to Grimestone's verses as well, of which nearly two-thirds are based on Latin models.[32] These normally appear on the same page close to the English renditions. The relation between Latin and English verses is of course of great importance for the history of the English religious lyric, and scholars have occasionally expressed uncertainty about which language is the original. As far as Grimestone's poems on death which appear in both languages are concerned, there can be little doubt that the respective Latin verses have claim to priority, because most of them are attested elsewhere without English translations and in manuscripts of earlier dates. Even where the monumental collection of medieval Latin verses of this kind, Hans Walther's *Proverbia sententiaeque latinitatis medii aevi,*[33] fails to list a Latin verse, it can be shown that Grimestone's English is translated from the Latin he quotes. A good example is No. 124, which reads thus:

> Alle we liuen hapfuliche,
> Noman ne trost wan he sal dey3e.
> Þerfore ne tak nouth wrongfuliche,
> For peraunter to-morwe þu gost þi wey3e.

The corresponding Latin passage is found in two hexameters:

> Viuimus hic sorte; noli spem ponere morte;
> Nil queras torte, morieris cras quia forte.[34]

[We live here by chance; do not put your trust in
death; do not seek anything wrongfully, because
perhaps tomorrow you will die.]

Here the metrical clumsiness of the English lines, when compared with the repeated rhyme sound of the leonine hexameters, would alone speak for the primacy of the Latin. Any remaining doubt is removed by the English word *hapfuliche*, which neatly translates *sorte* but, since it is not found elsewhere in Middle English writings, was evidently coined for this purpose.[35] In several cases these Latin source texts can be traced back to the eleventh century,[36] and one is actually put together from two classical authors.[37] But even where these sources and models are not clearly datable, it is quite safe to say that they belong to the enormous body of such material produced by clerical wits and preachers during the twelfth and thirteenth centuries.

This tradition of Latin *proverbia* and *sententiae* is, however, not the only source feeding into Friar Grimestone's lyrical output. Next to it is the learned tradition of preaching from which several of these lyrics stem even though they may not have exact source texts. Such is the English acrostic on D-E-T-H, which imitates similar acrostics on M-O-R-S.[38] Such is also a list of three properties of death, which could have been used as the division or *partitio* of a sermon:

> It is bitter to mannis mende;
> It is siker to mannis kende;
> It is delere of al our ende.[39]

[It is bitter to man's mind, it is assured to man's nature, it deals out the end to all of us.]

Such is, finally, a similar list of the Signs of Death, again a variant of a commonplace theme in medieval preaching, though its origins may well be English.[40] There are three other poems which have no Latin source in Grimestone's collection but are strongly reminiscent of Latin commonplaces or may have been inspired by a Latin quotation which Grimestone did not copy in his book. For instance, when Death exclaims

> Be war, man, I come as thef
> To reuen þi lif þat is þe lef,

[Beware, man, I come like a thief to rob your life that is dear to you],

one is at once reminded of half a dozen appropriate Bible passages,[41] though a medieval preacher may of course be trusted to have

possessed enough imagination to make a couplet on "death is a thief"
without having recourse to divine revelation.[42]

But a final half dozen verses clearly have a more popular, native
background. One is a proverb:

> On mo[r]ewe morwen comet al oure care
> Wan borwed ware wil hom fare;[43]

> [Tomorrow morning our worry will start, when bor-
> rowed goods want to go home.]

the second is similarly proverbial:

> With a sorwe and a clut
> Al þis werd comet in and out;[44]

> [With sorrow and a piece of cloth all this world
> comes in and out.]

and a third was in its entirety borrowed from *The Proverbs of Hending*.[45] The other three lyrics are of greater interest and will be
discussed in a moment. They are a version of the Visit to the Grave,
in two parts (i.e., a dialogue), and a version of the Earth-upon-
Earth poem.[46]

Whether Grimestone's lyrics on death stem from learned Latin
or from native traditions, it is evident that their form and substance
are thoroughly traditional, deriving from sources that reach back
to times long before the Black Death. And I should at once add
that the same is true of the thoughts they express, the attitudes they
reflect toward death. Here life appears as transient,[47] a borrowed
good which must be yielded up soon.[48] It begins and it ends in
sorrow.[49] Earthly riches and worldly pomp will profit nothing.[50]
Hence, we are asked not to defer doing good till tomorrow but to
think upon death.[51] Thus, the warning *Memento mori* is sounded
again and again in a number of imperatives: beware, have in mind,
seek, think, behold, do not trust![52] Death is certain to come, even
if we do not know its hour.[53] Neither prayer nor gifts can bring
us release.[54] With its advent, power and strength and beauty will
come to naught and all things will turn to dust.[55]

It would be tedious to document in detail these commonplace
thoughts and warnings, since they do not reflect new attitudes

evoked by the plague experience. Instead, we may single out for
comment one aspect of death lyrics which is often thought to have
been caused or at least intensified by the ravages of the plague:
their dwelling on the gruesome details of corpse and grave.
Grimestone does indeed offer three or four poems which share this
interest. One of his longer lyrics includes the following lines:

> þou he [i.e., man] be fair and strong in fith,
> To wirmes mete he sal ben dith.
> His faire eyne in þe heued sul senke,
> His gay bodi foul sal stinke.
> Þus solen we turnen child an man
> In puder of herde an be noman.[56]

> [Though man may be fair and strong in fight, he
> shall be prepared as food for worms. His fair eyes
> will sink into his head, his handsome body will give
> a foul stench. Thus will we, both child and grown
> man, turn to dust of earth and become nobody.]

The entire poem is translated from Latin, which has furnished the
references to worms and to the stench of the corpse.[57] One could,
however, detect an increased concern with gruesome details in the
fact that Grimestone expands those fairly bland references into very
precise and rhetorically pointed images, such as, "his fair eyes shall
sink into the head" and "his handsome body will give a foul stench,"
which are not found in his source. But I hesitate to see new attitudes in such minimal changes, especially since they too follow
older conventions of death poetry, realized particularly in the Body-
versus-Soul Debate and the Signs-of-Death traditions. The quoted
lines hardly illustrate the change effected by the Black Death which
some historians have seen in Western sensitivity during the fourteenth and fifteenth centuries, whereby an older concern with such
hideous details is said to have turned into an obsession.[58] The same
holds true for another poem, a warning directed to those who take
pride in clothing:

> þenk of þi cote þat is brith an gay,
> Hou it sal ben lined with grene an with g[ray].[59]

> [Think of your coat that is bright and gay, how it

will be lined with green and gray.]

Though the couplet is apparently not a direct translation, it was surely inspired by the biblical quotation that appears next to it (in Latin), taken from a chapter dealing with man's pride: "For when a man shall die, he shall inherit serpents" (Ecclesiasticus 10.13). Grimestone's couplet is unquestionably lively and shows poetic wit, but as unquestionably its sentiment goes all the way back to Ecclesiasticus. The hideousness of the corpse that appears in this and the previously quoted poem is a theme that was fully anticipated in *Fasciculus morum*, in both Latin and English.[60]

Another topic equally inspired Grimestone to some lines of his own invention, the Visit to the Grave.[61] This poem has been listed as two separate items, but these could easily be read as parts of a dialogue between a living and a dead person, in which each speaks four lines and each line of the stanza voiced by the living is echoed by the dead. In the manuscript the lines appear as follows:

> Her sal i duellen loken vnder ston,
> Her sal i duellen: ioye is her non.
> Her sal i duellen wermes to fede,
> Her sal i duellen domes to abide.

Si fas esset loqui, quilibet mortuus possit dicere "heu" propter quatuor:

> For i ham pore withouten frendes,
> In gret pine among þe fendis,
> Wirmis mete day an niht,
> To hard rekning I am dith.[62]

[Here shall I dwell, shut away under a stone. Here shall I dwell, where there is no joy. Here shall I dwell in order to feed worms. Here shall I dwell, to wait for my judgment. — If he were able to speak, any dead person could say "alas" for four reasons: For I am poor and without food; in great suffering among the fiends; worms' food day and night; and getting ready for a hard reckoning.]

The first quatrain is accompanied by four Latin lines (not hexameters), though it is not clear which of the two is the original.[63] But the second English stanza has no corresponding Latin: it is evidently modeled after the first English quatrain, whose images it repeats line by line. Both quatrains together represent, I think, a late version of native poems that formulate man's reflection on the grave, such as it was voiced much earlier in the beautiful thirteenth-century lyric "When the turf is thy tower" (which, incidentally, also appears in a collection made for preachers).[64]

Thus, even those Grimestone verses which speak of the hideousness of corpse and grave follow traditions that reach back to long before the Black Death. Whatever few indications of a new sentiment one may find in these poems seem to occur in the image of death as a personification. Rosemary Woolf has said that the personification itself, as it appears in the already quoted couplet, "Beware, man, I come like a thief," is a new development.[65] Beyond the literary device, one may detect in addition a new tone in the characterization of Death as a grim figure who stands and waits, who threatens, exacts, and brings misery.[66] The change can be found in Grimestone's translation of a Latin distich on the main topics of meditation:

> Mors tua, mors Domini, fraus mundi, gloria celi,
> Et dolor inferni sunt meditanda tibi.

> [Your death, the death of Our Lord, the world's
> deceit, heavenly glory, and the torment of hell —
> these are matters for you to meditate on.]

The distich exists in various forms in medieval Latin and was rendered in English rhyming lines as early as *Ancrene Wisse*. In contrast to his source and predecessors, Grimestone expands the bare *mors tua* into a whole line and renders it as "sorhfulhed of detȝ þat stant an waitet þe."[67] Similarly expanded characterizations of death appear in the following acrostic on D-E-T-H:

> Deth is a dredful dettour,
> Deth is an Elenge herbergour,
> Deth is a trewe tollere,
> And Deth is an hardi huntere.[68]

In comparison with the similar acrostic in *Fasciculus morum*, where

Death was likened to mirror, clock, thief, and summoner,
Grimestone uses images that are imbued with greater violence and
grimness, which are expressed in the properties themselves as well
as in the accompanying adjectives: fearful slayer (?),[69] loathsome
host (with the suggestion of lonesomeness and exile in *elenge*), truthful
(that is, exacting) toll-collector, and hardy (that is, stout or bold)
hunter.

As far as I can see, the foregoing consideration exhausts the
changes one finds in the representation of death in Grimestone's
poems when they are compared with earlier verses. It is very little, and I am not even certain that such minimal changes are really innovations. We are compelled to conclude that the preachers'
verses in Grimestone reveal no significant differences in their depiction of and attitude toward death from those written before 1350
and preserved in *Fasciculus morum* and other preaching aids. This
is true not only of the many short poems I have been considering
but also of the one extended lyric on death which appears in
Grimestone's book. It is a four-stanza poem which puns on the word
earth. Its first two stanzas read:

                    Herde maket halle,
                    And herde maket bour,
                    Herde reyset castel,
                    And herde reyset tour.

                    Wan herde is leyd in herde,
                    Blac is his bour.
                    Þan sal herde for herde
                    Hauen many a bitter sour.[70]

[Earth makes the hall, and earth makes the bower;
earth raises the castle, and earth raises the tower.
When earth is laid into earth, his bower is black;
then earth will have for earth many a bitter pang.]

This is not a bad poem, but its sentiment and punning technique
were anticipated, in more highly condensed form, in a well known
lyric "Erþe toc of erþe" preserved in MS. Harley 2253;[71] and the
very images of these two stanzas occur almost verbatim in a longer

poem on the same topic copied in another preachers' anthology that was made in the first quarter of the fourteenth century:

> Erþ bilt castles, and erþe bilt toures;
> Whan erþ is on erþe, blak beþ þe boures.[72]

Once again, I do not find that the plague experience has effected any change in Grimestone's lyrics on death.

At this point one might question the approach of this paper and ask whether I have not, after all, been looking at the wrong man. Was John Grimestone, perhaps, a stuffy old padre on whose lyrical style new trends and experiences simply would not make an impact? A look at his poems on topics other than death, however, quickly convinces us that this is not so at all. His lyrics on the Passion of Christ, for example — the other great topic that generated dozens and dozens of preachers' verses — contain some of the finest lyrical gems in Middle English and represent an astonishing poetic advance beyond the simple Passion verses in *Fasciculus morum* and similar collections.[73] In contrast to the short verses of earlier preaching manuals, many of Grimestone's Passion lyrics are long poems and songs composed in many stanzas;[74] rather than presenting simply a one-way appeal of the suffering Christ to mankind, they contain verses in which his appeal is answered either by man's response[75] or in a genuine dialogue with his mother.[76] In Grimestone's lyrics on the Passion there is the voice of a reflecting, meditative, loving "I", which produces a tone of intimacy that is completely lacking in earlier preachers' verses.[77] Finally, Grimestone also incorporates formal devices into his poems, such as dialogue,[78] the lullaby,[79] or the *pastourelle* opening,[80] which, although not new in English poetry, are innovations in verses that were destined for use in preaching. In his Passion lyrics (and we can add to them his lyrics on the Blessed Virgin) Grimestone goes far beyond *Fasciculus morum* towards a much greater lyricism.

But then, perhaps, the date at which Grimestone wrote his book (1372) is too early for the full impact of plague experience to show in English lyrics on death; perhaps one has to wait until the mid-fifteenth century for a more visible and powerful reflection of the successive plagues in lyric poetry. One cannot, of course, deny the numerical increase of macabre details in fifteenth-century death lyrics.[81] But it is also pertinent to recall the conclusion which Rosemary Woolf reached after meticulously investigating the sub-

ject and pursuing every apparently new image of poetic device:
"The English death lyric in the fifteenth century was surprisingly
unmeditative and . . . surprisingly limited in quantity and diffu-
sion. Judgments of size and quantity vary according to implicit
measures of comparison and the death lyric of the fifteenth century may, from the modern point of view, seem copious and
gruesome. But if it is measured against the contemporary French
production, then its scarcity is plain."[82] I would add that the same
impression of scarcity, drabness, and conventional rhetoric arises
when fifteenth-century English death lyrics are measured against
their precursors in the preaching books and collections of the fourteenth century. Individual poems may be longer and more elaborate,
but they do not explore new sentiments or invent new images; they
merely combine and recombine ancient commonplaces, and do so
more and more copiously.[83]

That the medieval plague experience left a surprisingly small and
unremarkable imprint on the artistic consciousness and imagination in England is true of other areas than the lyric as well. A good
example is that haunting motif which most readily comes to mind
when modern man thinks of the plague, the Dance of Death. Here
we find a succession of representatives of various social and professional classes, each led to death by a corpse or skeleton depicted
as dancing or playing a musical instrument. Originating either in
France or in Germany, the motif was extremely popular on the
Continent and has survived in countless visual representations there,
usually as paintings or woodcuts, as well as in verses that are alter-
nately spoken by Death and by such human types as pope, emperor,
queen, merchant, physician, cook, peasant, mother, and so forth.[84]
When one turns to England, one is surprised by the very small
number of representations of this kind of which we have any record
whatsoever, whether they have now disappeared or are still extant.[85]
Of the approximately one dozen relevant representations about
which enough details are known that allow us to form an accurate
picture, most are single scenes depicting only one living human
being and Death (shown as either a skeleton or a corpse). In many
cases these scenes seem to have nothing to do with the genuine
Dance of Death but instead represent different traditions that
originated before 1348, such as the *Vado mori,*[86] the Three Living
and the Three Dead,[87] or simply the Visit to the Grave or a similar
Memento mori.[88] Thus, the painting of "Death and the Gallant"
formerly seen in Salisbury Cathedral is more closely related to the

Visit-to-the-Grave tradition than to the Dance of Death, as the accompanying verses make clear;[89] and the pictures of a knight, king, and bishop being led off by Death that appear in fifteenth-century manuscripts illustrate, not a Dance of Death proper, but an English rendering of the *Vado mori.*[90] There are really only two visual works from medieval England about which we can be reasonably sure that they once contained a larger number of scenes such as we find in Continental Dances of Death: the panel paintings in Hexham Priory[91] and those at St. Paul's, London — and the latter were definitely modeled upon the famous set in the charnel house of Holy Innocents in Paris.[92]

One could go on and point to other forms of literature or the fine arts or even the liturgy[93] to demonstrate that in England the medieval plague experience has left a relatively insignificant impact on works of the imagination, if any at all. This is a disappointingly negative conclusion to our investigation, but it should be offered as a necessary corrective to the exaggerated and even rhapsodic statements about the influence of the Black Death on English art and literature and life in general that are sometimes made. It will not do, for instance, to say that "the popularity of the 'Danse Macabre' in England was never so great as in France" (which is true enough) and immediately continue to state that "there were numerous painted mural dances throughout the country," for which declaration there is simply no good evidence.[94] Or to quote a more recent remark about the bubonic plague in England: "This stark and recurrent catastrophe inevitably left its mark on the sensitivity of the time."[95] Maybe so, but in comparison with other themes and experiences, whatever mark has been left in concrete expressions in literature and the fine arts is not very visible.

Why should this have been the case? Short of postulating that the Black Death never happened in England, how can we explain this remarkable scarcity of artistic expressions of the medieval plague experience? To say with Rosemary Woolf that there was no "actual popular taste for literature on the subject of death" in fifteenth-century England[96] is of course merely begging the question. Her further suggestion that the taste for literary descriptions of death and the dying, of graves and corpses declined after the Black Death because the actual experience of these was so horrible and gruesome as to make their poetic representation unnecessary and undesired[97] is certainly worth considering; but it leaves unanswered the question why this should have been so in England while on the Continent the reverse was true.

One might suggest that the English, more than their Continental neighbors, realized that cheerfulness in the face of death is not only an excellent psychological defense but may actually have medicinal value. When Chaucer's Knight halts the Monk's interminable sequence of sad tales

for litel hevynesse
Is right ynough to muche folk, I gesse.
I seye for me, it is a greet disese,[98]

his attitude need not have been oriented by Lady Philosophy[99] but might reflect more down-to-earth medical views of the time. Notice that in one of the very few English poems that give practical advice against the plague John Lydgate recommends such cheerfulness as the very first preventive remedy:

Who will been holle and kepe hym fro sekenesse
And resiste the strok of pestilence,
Lat hym be glad, and voide al hevynesse.[100]

In further reflecting on the sparse impact left by the plague, I would also call attention to the essentially traditional and moralistic character which distinguishes late medieval English literature from its Continental counterparts. As the analysis of the Grimestone verses has shown, the experience of the Black Death and succeeding plagues cannot be credited with producing anything new in English lyrics on death. For additional demonstration I can point to a virtually unknown analogue to the Dance of Death which is preserved in a fifteenth-century manuscript written in England for English schoolboys. This is a Latin poem in 14 hexameters which, in dialogue form, has each of the seven deadly sins confronted by Death.[101] First the Vice characterizes itself briefly, and then Death remarks on the outcome of the Vice's actions in afterlife. Accidia or Sloth, for instance, says this:

Malo dormire quam Christi templa subire

[I would rather sleep than go to church.]

and Mors replies:

Non dormitabis quando penas tollerabis.

[You won't slumber when you suffer your
punishments!]

Here we find a sequence of presumably living characters, self-
characterization, and responses by Death that refer to a future
fate — all features which this poem shares with the Dance of Death.
But in place of representations from contemporary society this poem
uses the abstract personifications of the traditional chief sins; and
instead of satirizing the current estates[102] it repeats the age-old commonplaces of religious morality.

By the other aspect of late medieval English literature that I
mentioned — its moralistic character — I have in mind not so much
its moralizing tone as the tendency to link all phenomena to human
actions and behavior. Specifically, there seems to be no evidence
in English imaginative literature before 1500 that the plague experience awakened in a poet's mind a *theological* problem, an outcry perhaps that God is dead[103] or a self-conscious reflection that
at times people "would pray that the soul-slayer might give them
help in their collective distress."[104] Rather, the plague experience
invariably led to criticism of *moral* failures. We noticed earlier that
in *Piers Plowman* God's deafness to human petitions is justified as
a consequence of human pride and the friars' neglect to preach the
right things. Similarly, what is perhaps the finest Middle English
poem that carries a direct reference to the plague, the fifteenth-
century *Disputacioun betwyx the body and wormes*, not only utilizes traditional themes and motifs but also bears out the moralistic tendency I am speaking of in that the poem, through the debate form,
moves from the body's initial shock and horror and rebellion against
the worms feeding on it, to the insight that during life it had been
too proud of its beauty; and based on this recognition of moral
failure the body can in the end accept its fate and even come to
a reconciliation with its ghastly enemies: "Let vs kys and dwell to
gedyr euermore."[105]

Even Chaucer demonstrates this moralistic tendency. The story
told by his Pardoner concerns three young men who want to "sleen
this false traytour Deeth. / He shal be slayn, he that so manye
sleeth." They are roused to this enterprise by that moving description of "a privee theef men clepeth Deeth" who with his spear "hath

a thousand slayn this pestilence."[106] But the initial images of death and plague in this tale lead to no further exploration of the plague experience. Instead, the three protagonists die by dagger and rat poison, and their mutual slaughter is precisely motivated by their greed. Beyond this story itself, the entire *Pardoner's Prologue and Tale* deals explicitly with the sin of avarice, and no matter how modern readers may evaluate Chaucer's attitude towards the Pardoner, it is clearly the Pardoner's character, his moral identity, that occupies the center of the poet's attention. This preoccupation with man's moral universe is of course no obstacle to reaching the highest poetic achievement. I am only suggesting that it may explain the relatively insignificant impact which the Black Death had on Middle English literature, the mediocre as well as the best. If Langland and Gower and Chaucer had ever said, "the world is out of joint," they would not have thought of earthquakes and plagues *per se*, but rather of the moral disorders in the heart of man.

notes

1. Boccaccio, *Decameron*, "Introduzione."
2. Guillaume de Machaut, *Le Jugement dou Roy de Navarre*, ll. 347–458, following upon various other disasters; Ernest Hoepffner, ed., *Oeuvres de Guillaume de Machaut* (Paris, 1908), 1:149–53.
3. Francesco Petrarca, *Le Familiari*, 8.7, ed. Ugo Dotti, 1 vol. in 2 pts (Urbino, 1974), 1:872–83.
4. *PhysT*, 91; *MerT*, 1793; *Mel*, 1175; all Chaucer references are to F. N. Robinson, ed., *The Works of Geoffrey Chaucer*, 2d ed. (Boston, 1957).
5. *WBT*, 1263–64. The other occurrences in oaths are: *NPT*, 3410; *MerT*, 2252–53. The remaining three references to the plague are at *GP*, 442 (the Physician "kepte that he wan in pestilence"), *KniT*, 2469 (Saturn causes pestilence), and *PardT*, 679 (see below).
6. *Piers Plowman*, C.I,82. I follow the C-text and silently imply that the reference also appears in A (when applicable) and B unless otherwise in-

dicated, and I quote from the edition by Walter W. Skeat, *The Vision of William concerning Piers the Plowman, in Three Parallel Texts*, 2 vols. (Oxford, 1886).

7. C.XI, 272-73.

8. C.XII, 55 ff.

9. C.VI, 114-16.

10. C.IX, 549-50 (only in C); my translation.

11. C.XXIII, 95-105; my translation.

12. C.XII, 60-62 (not in A); my translation.

13. C.XVI, 217-29; my translation.

14. *Mum and the Sothsegger*, M, l. 1369; ed. Mabel Day and Robert Steele, *EETS* 199 (London, 1936), p. 66.

15. The poem "A Warning to be ware," in the Vernon MS, discusses the rising of the Commons of 1381, the earthquake of 1382, and the pestilence; only the first two are described at some length; see F. J. Furnivall, ed., *The Minor Poems of the Vernon MS*, vol. 2, *EETS* 117 (London, 1901), pp. 719-21; the pestilence is mentioned in l. 58. Margery Kempe mentions *pestylens* in a series of tribulations and warnings sent by God, but also refers to a particular occurrence of the plague; see *The Book of Margery Kempe*, Sanford Brown Meech and Hope Emily Allen, eds., *EETS* 212 (London, 1940), pp. 48, 185, 202, and 337, n. to 202/16. *The Pricke of Conscience* mentions pestilences in a series of disasters, but this is a translation of Luke 21:11; see the edition by Richard Morris (1863; reprint ed., New York, 1973), p. 110, l. 4035. Gower has a similar series in Latin, which seems indebted to the same biblical prophecy: *Vox clamantis*, 7:22; ed. G. C. Macaulay, *The Complete Works of John Gower* (Oxford, 1902), 4:305. My quotation in the text comes from Woodburn O. Ross, ed., *Middle English Sermons*, *EETS* 209 (London, 1960), p. 312, from a MS copied around 1450.

16. Priscilla Heath Barnum, ed., *Dives and Pauper*, *EETS* 275 (London, 1976). The following references are to this edition, by part, chapter, and page. This volume comprises only the first half of the work. In the remainder of the treatise, *moreyn* appears only once again, but refers to an epidemy among animals. I have consulted the reprint of Pynson's editon of 1493, prepared with an introduction and index by Francis J. Sheeran (Delmar, N.Y., 1973); the reference is in IX.ix.

17. I,xvii, pp. 117-18; I,xx, p. 125; I,xxvii, p. 143; I,xxix, p. 149 (the comet of 1402); I,xxxi, p. 152 (evil spirits may cause *moreyn* and other disasters.)

18. I,xxviii, pp. 146-47; my translation.

19. I,xlvii, p. 183, on the belief that the first day of the year indicates what will befall later.

20. I,xlii, p. 170; my translation. *Moreyn* occurs again in I,lii, p. 192, with other disasters of biblical times.

21. Rosemary Woolf, *The English Religious Lyric in the Middle Ages* (Oxford, 1968), pp. 373-374. To her examples must be added the sermon

collection made by Bishop John Sheppey, O.S.B., in MS. Merton College, Oxford, 248.
22. On these "preachers' tags" see S. Wenzel, *Verses in Sermons. "Fasciculus Morum" and Its Middle English Poems* (Cambridge, Mass., 1978), especially chapter 2.
23. See Edward Wilson, *A Descriptive Index of the English Lyrics in John of Grimestone's Preaching Book*, Medium Aevum Monographs, n.s., 2 (Oxford, 1973).
24. The subject index at the beginning of the manuscript lists 143 numbered topics, but the last three are missing in the codex, which seems incomplete.
25. Seven of these are duplicates in this manuscript; see Wilson, *A Descriptive Index*, p. xi.
26. A full description of the work, its date, and the English verses it contains can be found in *Verses in Sermons*.
27. The chapter *De memoria mortis* appears in Bodleian Library, MS. Rawlinson C.670, fols. 20v–121v, from which I have translated these excerpts. I have added translations of the Middle English and Latin verses and have identified biblical quotations, all in square brackets; for the translations of biblical verses I have used the Douai version. For a critical edition of the English verses see *Verses in Sermons*, pp. 148–53.
28. Edinburgh, Advocates MS. 18.7.21, fols. 86r–87v. Notice that although death was a favorite topic in fourteenth-century preaching, the section devoted to it in Grimestone is shorter than those on prayer, obedience, Christ's Passion, and others.
29. Wilson, nos. 109–130.
30. Wilson, nos. 53 (verse translation of Rom. 8:13); 138 (topics for meditation); 225 (on pride of clothes); 226 ("Unde superbis homo?"); 228 ("Vide qualis eris"); 239 (Three Sorrowful Things). There are of course others that refer to death, but they do not make it their central concern.
31. The death poems that here occur outside the chapter *De memoria mortis* include such verses on mortality as a translation of "Unde superbis, homo" and the "Signs of Death," nos. 4239 and 4035 in Carleton Brown and Rossell Hope Robbins, *The Index of Middle English Verse* (New York, 1942), henceforth referred to as *Index*. Both have been often printed.
32. Translated from biblical quotations are Wilson, nos. 53, 109, 119; from Latin verses, Wilson, nos. 113, 115, 118, 121–26, 138, 226, 228, 239; no. 120, a stanza from *The Proverbs of Hending*, with its last line "þe ex is at þe rote," evidently came to Grimestone's mind through Matt. 3:10, which is quoted before it. No. 128 has a Latin equivalent next to it, but may be originally English; it goes with no. 129, which will be discussed later. No. 225, also discussed below, may have been inspired by Eccles. 10:13.
33. Six volumes, including a Register (Göttingen, 1963–69), henceforth referred to as Walther, *Proverbia*.
34. MS. Advocates 18.7.21, fol. 87v. Wilson prints only the first line of the Latin, a practice followed throughout his descriptive index. I was

able to examine the manuscript thanks to a grant from the American Philosophical Society and the good services of Miss Yeo of the National Library of Scotland.

35. It is not listed in the *Middle English Dictionary*. Compare also the translation of "pellis et ossa" as "sken and bon," in no. 122. If this were a truly native poem, one would expect to find "fles and fel."

36. For instance, Wilson, no. 115: its Latin source (Walther, *Proverbia*, 25516) is attested from the eleventh century onward. Similarly the Latin of nos. 123 and 226 goes back at least to the twelfth century.

37. Wilson, no. 113; the two Latin hexameters derive from Lucan and Ovid respectively: see Walther, *Proverbia*, 17080b (and 27978) and 24398.

38. Wilson, no. 112, quoted and further discussed below. For the Latin counterpart, see the discussion of *Fasciculus morum*, above, p. 138.

39. Wilson, no. 111.

40. Wilson, no. 127. For the topic and its tradition, see Rossell Hope Robbins, "Signs of Death in Middle English," *Mediaeval Studies* 32 (1970): 282–98, esp. 295. His footnote 43 needs correction: the ten verses referred to appear on fol. 87 verso; the quatrain "Wat so þu art" is on 87 recto (with eight more verses), and the heading *De morte* appears fol. 86r.

41. Wilson, no. 110. *Cf.* Job 24:14; Matt. 24:43; Luke 12:39; 1 Thess. 5:2; 2 Pet. 3:10; Rev. 16:15. See also the image of death as a *raptor rapiens* in the Latin acrostic of *Fasciculus morum* quoted earlier, and similar images in many Latin verses, such as Walther, *Proverbia*, 15171a ("venit occulto more latronis"), 15194c-d, 15195, 15195a-b, etc.

42. The other two poems that are possibly inspired by a Latin model are no. 114 (which may derive from the distich "Cornicis more cras est tibi semper in ore . . ." written next to it) and no. 225, discussed below.

43. Wilson, no. 117; *cf.* Bartlett Jere Whiting and Helen Wescott Whiting, *Proverbs, Sentences, and Proverbial Phrases from English Writings Mainly before 1500* (Cambridge, Mass., 1968), T.108 and G.71, on "Borrowed thing will home again" and "borrowed ware."

44. Wilson, no. 116.

45. Wilson, no. 120. *Cf.* stanza 39 in the edition by G. Schleich, "Die Sprichwörter Hendings und die Prouerbis of Wysdom," *Anglia* 51 (1927): 268–69. The stanza also appears separately in MS. Royal 8.E.xvii and in the late thirteenth-century treatise on the vices used in Chaucer's *Parson's Tale*; see S. Wenzel, "Unrecorded Middle English Verses," *Anglia* 92 (1974): 69, no. 51.

46. Wilson, nos. 128–29 and 130, respectively.

47. Wilson, nos. 109 and 123.

48. *Cf.* Wilson, no. 117.

49. *Cf.* Wilson, nos. 116 and 226.

50. *Cf.* Wilson, no. 122.

51. *Cf.* nos. 113, 114, and 121.

52. *Cf.* nos. 110, 119, 120, 124, 225, and 228.

53. *Cf.* nos. 111, 125, and 239.

54. *Cf.* no. 118.

55. *Cf.* nos. 126, 130, 225, 226, and 228.

56. Wilson, no. 226, ll. 7–12.

57. Wilson fails to cite the Latin: "Unde superbit homo cuius conceptio culpa . . .;" see Walther, *Proverbia*, 32163, a very popular distich found from the twelfth century onward. Grimestone has three distichs, the last clearly serving as the model for the quoted English lines:

Post hominem vermis, post vermem fetor et horror.
Sic in non-hominem vertitur omnis homo.

[After man comes the worm, after the worm stench and horror. Thus every man is turned into noman.] This final distich is Walther, *Proverbia*, 22006, likewise attested from the twelfth century onward.

58. "Death had always been a preoccupation of medieval man; now it became an obsession." Philip Ziegler, *The Black Death* (New York, 1969), p. 132. Similarly, Philippa Tristram speaks of "tendencies which the Black Death does not initiate, but which it certainly brings into prominence, and even renders into obsessions"; *Figures of Life and Death in Medieval English Literature* (New York, 1976), p. 13.

59. Wilson, no. 225. For the connection of death with "green," which puzzled Wilson, see W. Heuser, ed., *Die Kildare-Gedichte, Bonner Beiträge zur Anglistik* 14 (Bonn, 1904): p. 182: "Whan erþ makiþ is liuerei, he graueþ vs in grene" (stanza 5 of *Index* 3939); and Robbins, "Signs of Death," p. 295: "Qwhen þi here is waxin grene" (l. 3 of *Supplement* 4049.7). See also *Supplement* 4049.6, printed by Karl Brunner, "Mittelenglische Todesgedichte," *Archiv* 167 (1935): 30.

60. See the (Latin) quotation attributed to St. Bernard and the English verse, "Was þer neuer caren so lothe" (*Index* 2283), quoted above, p. 136. For Old English passages on the signs of corruption, see Woolf, *English Religious Lyric*, pp. 94–95.

61. For the topic see Woolf, ibid., pp. 88–89 and 401–4. Grimestone has two more poems on this topic ("Sum quod eris"), nos. 115 and 228, both spoken by the dead person, but they are rather colorless and translate Latin verses.

62. Wilson, nos. 128–29. The verbal form of these lines suggests that they were intended as a division.

63. "Hic habitabo clausus in tumulo . . . ," with end-rhyme aabb. Robbins, *Supplement* 1210.5, believes the English to be a translation, but Woolf doubts that (*English Religious Lyrics*, p. 88, n. 3), and I tend to agree with her. The phrase "loken under ston" certainly has a native ring to it.

64. *Index* 4044. For a discussion of this collection, see Karl Reichl, *Religiöse Dichtung im englischen Hochmittelalter* (Munich, 1973). See also *Index* 4119, another poem found in the same thirteenth-century manuscript, which has many very precise gruesome details indeed (printed in Reichl, p. 88).

65. Woolf, *English Religious Lyric*, pp. 336–37.

66. For a succinct but incisive analysis of various fourteenth- and

fifteenth-century representations of Death see the sensitive study by Alberto Tenenti, *La vie et la mort à travers l'art du XVe siècle* (Paris, 1952).

67. Wilson, no. 138. The version in *Ancrene Wisse* is *Index* 3568. It merely states, "þench of þin ahne deað."

68. Wilson, no. 112.

69. I am puzzled by the first line of this poem. At first glance it seems to mean, "Death is a fearsome debtor," but this makes no sense because, while mankind owes death as a debt to nature or to God, death cannot be called debtor, least of all in a sequence of agent nouns such as occur here; *creditor* would be more appropriate. The same semantic problem exists in *The Castle of Perseverance*, l. 2821, where Death says, "But whane I dele my derne dette" (Mark Eccles, ed., *The Macro Plays*, *EETS* 262 [London, 1969], p. 86). One might postulate a Middle English noun *dette* with the agent noun *dettour*; the word could be related to Old English *dyttan*, Middle English *ditten/dutten*, "to close, enclose," which was used with the denotation of "to bury." But more probably it is related to Middle Dutch *dutten* (II), "to strike a blow"; see *Woordenboek der Nederlandsche Taal*, III.2 ('s-Gravenhage, 1916), col. 3681.

70. Wilson, no. 130. Wilson suggests the reading *stour* for *sour*, but no emendation is needed if one takes the word to mean *shower*, which mades good sense (see *OED*, s.v. *Shower*, sb.1, 5) and agrees with Grimestone's habit of occasionally representing initial *sh-* as *s-* (*sort, scrud, sal, solen*, etc.).

71. Listed in *Index* as 3939, which gives the wrong impression that the Harley poem is a fragment of the Kildare poem.

72. *Kildare-Gedichte*, p. 182, st. 6; *Index* 3939. For the tradition of such "Earth-upon-Earth" poems, see Hilda M. R. Murray, ed., *The Middle English Poem, Erthe upon Erthe*, *EETS* 141 (London, 1911).

73. In the following notes, I will simply cite some representative examples without any attempt at being exhaustive. I choose examples from Carleton Brown, ed., *Religious Lyrics of the XIVth Century*, second edition, revised by G. V. Smithers (Oxford, 1952), and refer to them as *RL XIV* and their respective numbers.

74. *RL XIV*, nos. 66 (three stanzas), 67 (36 lines), 69 (24 lines plus burden), 72 (36 lines).

75. *RL XIV*, no. 68.

76. *RL XIV*, no. 67; also 75.

77. *RL XIV*, nos. 68, 69, 71.

78. *RL XIV*, nos. 56, 67, 75.

79. *RL XIV*, nos. 56, 59, 65.

80. *RL XIV*, nos. 56, 58.

81. For a good example, see the poem printed by Woolf, *English Religious Lyric*, pp. 318-19.

82. Ibid., pp. 352-53.

83. As Woolf puts it: Fifteenth-century death lyrics achieve length and elaboration "by the spreading of earlier material more thinly" (ibid., p. 309). See also Tristram, *Figures of Life and Death*, p. 172.

84. The best recent study, with a very rich bibliography, is Hellmut Rosenfeld, *Der mittelalterliche Totentanz*, 3d ed. (Köln/Wien, 1974), even though some of its views about its (German) origins are not universally accepted.

85. James M. Clark, *The Dance of Death in the Middle Ages and the Renaissance* (Glasgow, 1950), chap. 2, gives a good survey of the relevant monuments in Great Britain. See also the slightly different list in Rosenfeld, *Totentanz*, p. 353, and a description of extant works by Ethel C. Williams, "The Dance of Death in Painting and Sculpture in the Middle Ages," *Journal of the British Archaeological Association*, 3d. ser., 1 (1937): 237–39.

86. The *Vado-mori* poem, its history, and its differences from the Dance of Death proper, is fully discussed by Rosenfeld, *Totentanz*, chap. 2 and passim. See also Eleanor P. Hammond, "Latin Texts of the Dance of Death," *MP* 8 (1910–11), 399–410, who does not draw as clear a distinction as Rosenfeld.

87. See the full analysis by Willy Rotzler, *Die Begegnung der drei Lebenden und der drei Toten* (Winterthur, 1961), with a selective bibliography of the more important older investigations on pp. 275–76.

88. All these different conventions and forms are briefly discussed by Woolf, *English Religious Lyric*, chaps. 3 and 9 and app. H. Similarly, Douglas Gray, *Themes and Images in the Medieval English Religious Lyric* (London, 1972), chap. 10.

89. *Cf.* the final line: "For such as they are such shalt thou be," printed by Francis Douce, *The Dance of Death exhibited in elegant engravings on wood* . . . (London, 1833), pp. 52–53, with a reproduction of a print made of the painting in 1748. My point can also be argued from the visual details of the painting: the figure of Death does not dance and does not lead the young man off.

90. See Karl Brunner, "Mittelenglische Todesgedichte," *Archiv* 167 (1935): 20–22. Two manuscript pages with illustrations are reproduced in Gray, *Themes and Images*, plates 10 (with figures of Death) and 11 (without such figures).

91. Clark, *Dance of Death*, pp. 7–8 and plate.

92. Ibid., pp. 11–13. The paintings were apparently connected with John Lydgate's poem *The Dance Macabre*, translated from the French verses he had seen in Paris. See E. P. Hammond, *English Verse between Chaucer and Surrey* (1927; reprint ed., New York, 1969), pp. 124–42 and 418–35; and Florence Warren and Beatrice White, eds., *The Dance of Death, EETS* 181 (London, 1931).

93. For example, there is very little evidence that the "plague saints" Sebastian and Roch enjoyed much popularity in England.

94. Beatrice White, in Warren and White, *The Dance of Death*, p. xviii.

95. Tristram, *Figures of Life and Death*, p. 8.

96. Woolf, *English Religious Lyric*, p. 353.

97. Ibid., pp. 310–11; similarly, Tristram, *Figures of Life and Death*, pp. 181–82.

98. *Canterbury Tales*, VII.2769–71.

99. As was suggested by Robert E. Kaske, "The Knight's Interruption of the *Monk's Tale*," *ELH* 24 (1957): 249–68.

100. John Lydgate, "A Doctrine for Pestilence," ll. 1–3, in Henry Noble MacCracken, ed. *The Minor Poems of John Lydgate, EETS* 192 (London, 1934), pt. 2, p. 702.

101. In British Library, Additional MS 37075, fol. 274v, a large fifteenth-century collection of grammatical treatises, vocabularies, proverbs, and much else, in Latin, French, and English. For a description of the volume, see *Catalogue of Additions to the MSS in the British Museum, 1900–1905* (London, 1907), pp. 344–49. The poem under discussion is Item 34. In contrast to the *Catalogue*, I read its first line as "Scandens ut luna sum cunctis altior una," which is more appropriate to Pride than "splendens" and of course agrees with "scandis" in line 2. The poem seems to be unique and is not listed by Walther, *Proverbia* and *Initia*, nor by Morton W. Bloomfield, B.-G. Guyot, D. R. Howard, and T. B. Kabealo, *Incipits of Latin Works on the Vices and Virtues, 1100–1500 A.D.* (Cambridge, Mass., 1979).

102. The Dance of Death as a vehicle for estates criticism and satire is discussed by Rosenfeld, *Totentanz*, pp. 137–39, 201–3, 275–76, and 300.

103. "God is dead" actually occurs as a line in a popular complaint poem beginning "Might is right" (*Index* 2167) which seemingly dates from the middle of the fourteenth century but is not connected with the plague.

104. Friedrich Klaeber, ed., *Beowulf*, ll. 176–78; my translation. Although there may well have been instances of devil worship in England in consequence of the plagues, I know of no evidence. There was a similar absence of other forms of social paranoia that occurred on the Continent, such as the flagellants or persecution of Jews and "semeurs de la peste."

105. The poem (*Index* 1563) was printed by Brunner, "Mittelenglische Todesgedichte," pp. 29–35, and has been discussed by Woolf, *English Religious Lyric*, pp. 328–30, and with even greater penetration by Klaus Jankofsky, "A View into the Grave: 'A Disputacion betwyx þe Body and Wormes' in British Museum MS Add. 37049," *TAIUS* 1 (1974): 137–59.

106. *Canterbury Tales*, VI.699–700 and 675–79.

The Black Death includes six incisive studies of the great pestilence of 1348 and its aftershocks. The Introduction by Nancy Siraisi describes the present state of the major questions surrounding the Black Death, from the reliability of casualty estimates to the responses of the intellectual elite. A demographic update by J. M. W. Bean introduces new English evidence for bubonic and pneumonic fatalities through the late fourteenth century. Aldo Bernardo argues that the plague, far from being mere stage scenery for the *Decameron*, must be understood as a condition of Boccaccio's message, while Divine providence in the mass mortality is the concern of Michael Dols' study, in a Moslem context. Joseph Polzer relocates certain peculiar forms of "plague iconography" in the decades preceding 1348; and Siegfried Wenzel scrutinizes English literary sensibilities for signs of bubonic morbidity. Robert Lerner discusses eschatological prophecies and ways in which the plague figured in an eschatological framework.

Daniel Williman is Assistant Professor of Classical and Near Eastern Studies at the State University of New York at Binghamton.